Livwise

easy recipes for a healthy, happy life

Olivia Newton-John

MURDOCH BOOKS

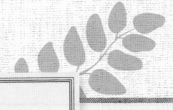

Contents

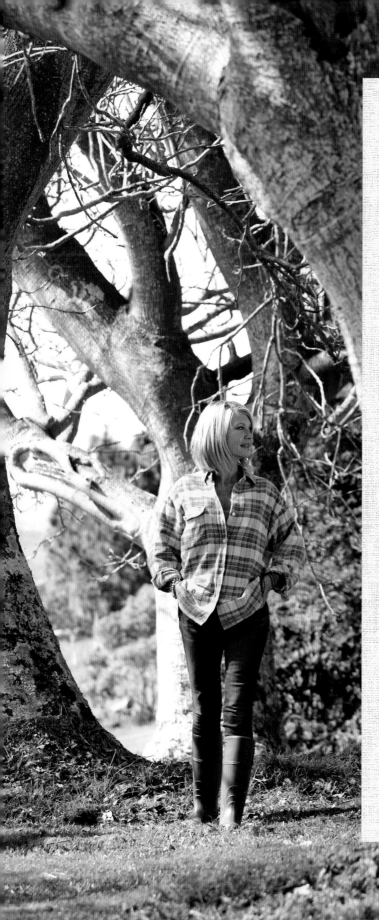

introduction

This is my first book — ever! Who would have thought it would be a cookbook? Over my lifetime I have made two attempts at writing a book but didn't finish either of them. This book means more to me than my previous attempts as it isn't about my personal life, but my life experience with food, the effect it has on my body and how eating the right foods in combination has helped to keep me fit and healthy.

There is an old, familiar saying 'We are what we eat!' and I am a firm believer that what we put into our bodies creates the building blocks of our existence. I also believe that what we think about what we eat is just as important. Considering where food is grown, how it is transported and stored, and finally, how it is prepared, means that each meal can be gratefully received and enjoyed as the precious gift that it is. Every plant and animal once had life, and each time I eat, I try to acknowledge this and honour that life with a quiet grace.

There are thousands of cookbooks on the market but what makes this one so special is not just my own passion for the role food has in maintaining good health, but the support I have had in compiling the recipes. I have been fortunate to be able to include recipes written by some of my favourite people, whose taste buds I respect. The contributors in this book have not only devoted their time, but also their knowledge of food and experience in the kitchen to ensure that this collection of recipes not only reflects the way I like to eat, but may help set you on the path to a healthier lifestyle.

Naturally, my first port of call was to all the talented chefs, both past and present, at Gaia Retreat and Spa in Byron Bay, Australia (www.gaiaretreat.com.au) — which in my opinion is the best healing retreat in the world, and my favourite place to eat. As co-owner, I was proud to develop an organic garden at the retreat so that the food we serve can be picked fresh each day — just a part of what makes mealtimes at Gaia so special.

Karen Inge, a well-respected nutritionist from Melbourne, Australia, was also asked to contribute to *LivWise*. I have been lucky enough to dine at Karen's table and her food is always delicious, nutritious and beautiful to behold!

In early 2010 I was in Australia fundraising for The Olivia Newton-John Cancer and Wellness Centre (ONJCWC) and someone gave me a book to read called *From Cancer to Wellness: The Forgotten Secrets*. I couldn't put it down. It was written by Kristine Matheson, also a cancer thriver, who, as coincidence would have it, lives very close to Gaia Retreat. I was so impressed with her book and her thoughts on raw food that I immediately asked if she would contribute some of her recipes and she kindly has.

The common thread between all these recipes is the food philosophy behind them and a mutual respect for the importance of eating a healthy balanced diet and increasing your intake of plant foods, some raw as well as organic foods where possible. Along with regular exercise, this helps your body find its own natural balance and achieve a healthy weight. The aim of this book therefore is to introduce you to ways of eating that will help to keep you in good health, whether you are going through the cancer journey or just wanting to maintain optimum health.

We have included many tasty simple vegetarian meals within these covers. You can add fish or meat as you wish, but I'm always pleasantly surprised at how satisfying vegetarian meals can be on their own. We all agree that you have to enjoy what you eat, so there are also sweet treats included.

I am very proud to say that 100 per cent of the profits I receive from the sale of *LivWise* will support the Olivia Newton-John Cancer and Wellness Centre (www.oliviaappeal.com) to help make available cutting-edge treatments and support cancer research. I am proud to say it will include a dedicated Wellness Centre with complimentary programs, such as massage, yoga and music therapy and so much more, that focus on the needs of the whole person — body, mind and spirit. It is a centre I dreamed of as I was going through my cancer journey. Ultimately, my vision is that cancer becomes a footnote in history.

Love and light,
Olivia

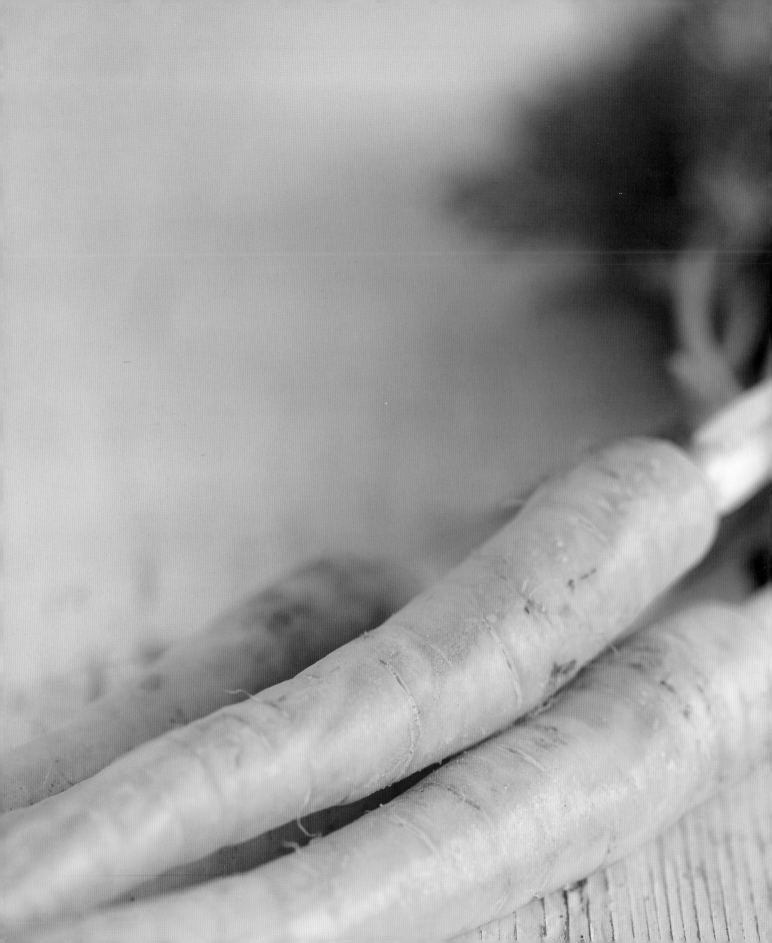

the common sense diet

Now that I am eighteen years past my initial diagnosis of breast cancer and feeling better than I've ever felt before I think of myself as a cancer thriver! People often ask me what my secret is and want to know how I manage to stay slim, active and healthy at my age — I feel timeless and even though my passport says so it is hard for me to comprehend that I am 62 years young!

I am no cordon bleu chef, nor am I a doctor or nutritionist, but I have picked up some pieces of information over the years about health and nutrition. Without getting too complicated, I wanted to present in this book some of what I do to stay healthy.

As I sat down to write this book I began to realise how many different eating choices I have succumbed to over the years. I have been a vegetarian at times, followed a strict macrobiotic diet on occasion, restricted my dairy and wheat intake on and off and have now returned to a more balanced diet that includes chicken and fish and occasionally some red meat. I am a very simple cook and like to keep things pretty basic in the kitchen (thanks Mum!). I believe first and foremost that simplicity is the key to healthy eating. I love eating this way as I can taste the freshness of my food. To me it seems obvious — when I start adding heavy sauces and toppings to meals I get into trouble!

The simplest way for me to explain my food philosophy is to remember that what goes up must come down. What you eat goes in, and if it doesn't come out it has to go somewhere else — like on your hips! I believe it starts with a combination of controlling the portion size of what goes in, ensuring the food is of the best quality you can find (organic is preferable), exercising regularly, drinking lots of water, and eating enough fibre to keep your internal wheels turning so you can expel the waste, and any toxins, efficiently.

Of course, following a diet can be hard to do over long periods of time. I am lucky I have a quick metabolism and I listen to my body. If I eat a large amount of food one day, the next day my body will tell me to ease up. I cut back on my food intake and do a work-out. That way, I never let my body accrue extra kilograms.

From what I have learned over the years the one thing that everybody seems to agree upon is that combining a balanced diet with regular exercise and clean water (and, I believe, a positive attitude) is the best-known way to stay healthy. A balanced diet should consist mostly of plants, vegetables and fruit, some wholegrains, nuts and seeds. It should include some protein-rich foods such as fish, poultry, eggs, dairy, legumes (beans and lentils) and a small amount of healthy fats, such as avocados, nuts, seeds and seed oils, olive oil and oily fish.

This is basically the eating regime I follow. It's not really a secret at all. I call it the common sense diet!

listen to your instincts

In all areas of my life I have learned to trust my instincts — after all, they once saved my life. After finding a lump in my breast (it wasn't the first, but all the others had been benign) I went to the doctor to have it checked. I was sent for a mammogram, which was negative. I then had a needle biopsy, which also turned out to be negative. I still wasn't feeling right in myself or with the lump, which was a little tender, so my doctor and I decided I should undergo some exploratory surgery. Although I had heard that breast cancer wasn't necessarily tender to the touch, this was my experience, and I'm glad I listened to my instincts and persevered.

In the end they found that the lump in my breast was cancerous. The cancer was removed, I had reconstructive surgery and underwent chemotherapy for about eight months. I have yearly mammograms now, and although the medical term used is 'remission', I don't like that word; it sounds like the cancer is lurking — I say it's gone! I tell this story not to scare women but to encourage them to do regular self-breast examinations and to trust themselves and their instincts if they feel something isn't right. (For more detailed information about how to do this yourself you can download a copy of a step-by-step breast self exam on my website www.liv.com.)

This experience reinforced the general idea that listening to your body and being conscious of the role nutrition can play in decreasing the risk of disease and helping to restore your body to its natural state of balance is so important.

After my experience with breast cancer I became even more conscious of what I was eating and tried the macrobiotic diet of Michio Kushi, one of the early leaders of the macrobiotic movement. I had heard that a macrobiotic diet was very cleansing and gave the body a chance to heal itself. In a nutshell, macrobiotics is all about eating food that is as natural as possible and avoiding foods that have been highly processed and refined. At the time I was eating a low-fat, high-fibre diet that did not include any meat, dairy products or sugar. A macrobiotic diet typically consists of about 60 per cent wholegrains, 30 per cent vegetables (it encourages you to eat these raw where possible) and the remaining 10 per cent is made up of bean and bean products, such as tempeh and tofu. It encourages people to eat some fruits and consume nuts and seeds in moderation while at the same time places emphasis on eating food grown locally and in season.

When I was going through treatment I employed a chef for a few months to cook my macrobiotic meals. I eventually eased my way out of the rigidity of the diet but learnt to respect much of its philosophy.

Luckily my mother, Irene, who was born and raised in Germany, set great food examples for me when I was a child. She fed me healthy food — rye and pumpernickel bread instead of white bread sandwiches in my lunchbox and dinners that almost always consisted of steamed potatoes (skins included), steamed broccoli and carrot. We ate plenty of fresh salads, delicious dishes of red cabbage made the German way with apple, and steamed or baked chicken breast or fish. For dessert we would have baked apples, pears or whatever fruit was in season, topped with a dollop of yoghurt. Mum would often make her own yoghurt, and always insisted that it was terrific for our digestive systems and she was right — probiotic yoghurt (the kind that contains health-promoting live bacteria) is still a favourite of mine.

It was all very simple and basic cooking, and while I was annoyed at the time that I wasn't able

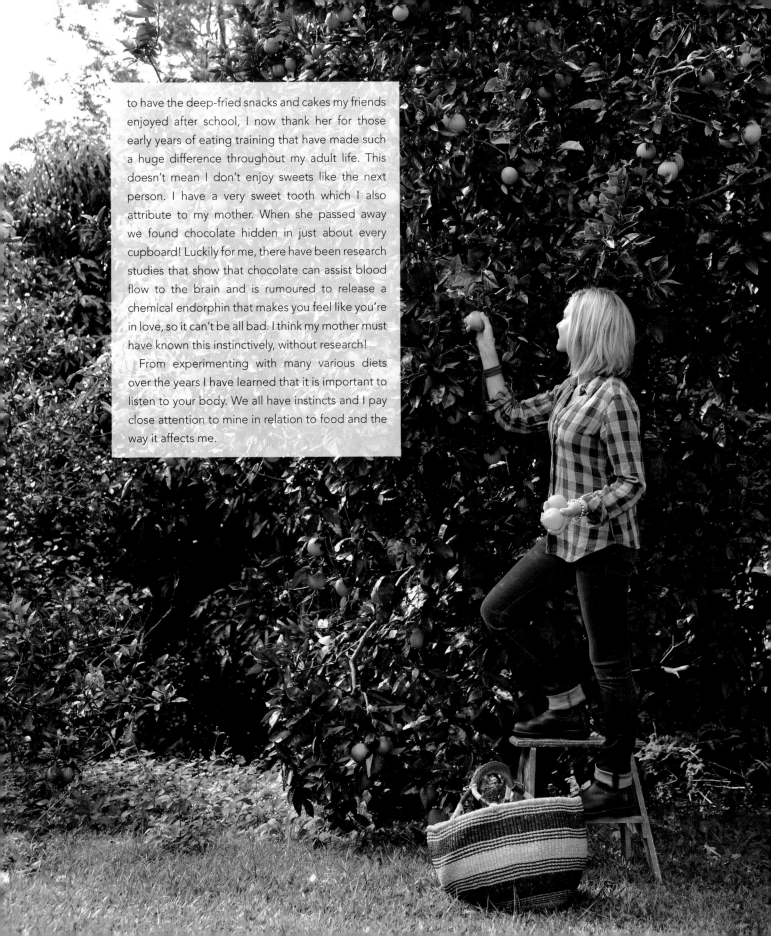

to have the deep-fried snacks and cakes my friends enjoyed after school, I now thank her for those early years of eating training that have made such a huge difference throughout my adult life. This doesn't mean I don't enjoy sweets like the next person. I have a very sweet tooth which I also attribute to my mother. When she passed away we found chocolate hidden in just about every cupboard! Luckily for me, there have been research studies that show that chocolate can assist blood flow to the brain and is rumoured to release a chemical endorphin that makes you feel like you're in love, so it can't be all bad. I think my mother must have known this instinctively, without research!

From experimenting with many various diets over the years I have learned that it is important to listen to your body. We all have instincts and I pay close attention to mine in relation to food and the way it affects me.

LivWise organically

I always look for, and try to buy, organically. Organic food contains fewer pesticides and toxins. It is my belief that eating organically as much as possible really does make a difference to our overall health.

There are countless pesticides used in the cultivation of mass-produced fruit and vegetables, most of which have never been tested on humans. This is an issue that I became very involved with when my dear friends, Nancy and Jim Chuda, lost their five-year-old daughter, Colette, to Wilms Tumour — a kidney cancer that is believed to be environmentally caused. She was my daughter Chloe's best friend and it was a heartbreaking experience for us all. The Chuda's incredible spirit and their strong Buddhist faith helped them create something positive out of their pain, an organisation called Healthy Child Healthy World (www.healthychild.org) to inform parents of the toxins that their children are exposed to in their everyday environment, including the chemicals found in food. I am proud to say that the organisation is now aligned with webmd.com, the most respected online source of medical information in the world.

Buying organically supports the organic produce industry and our spending dollars can effect change and increase the demand for organically grown food. I also try to buy locally grown — it is bound to be fresher, taste better, and saves the fossil costs of storage and transportation. Most importantly though, seeking out organic produce means you are not ingesting the pesticides that are still allowed to contaminate some of our foods and products.

As I like to limit my exposure to chemicals as much as I possibly can — at least to the ones I know about — I am pleased to see that most supermarkets are now carrying a variety of organic foods, fruits and vegetables.

anti what?

It has taken a few years of trial and error to find the diet that suits my body best, but the recipes in this cookbook represent the kinds of foods I now love to eat (some cooked and some raw), and they are tasty, healthy and delicious too!

I have done a lot of reading about diets and words like 'antioxidant' keep cropping up. 'Antioxidant' is a word I see everywhere. For a while I never really understood what it meant, but was too embarrassed to admit it!

I remember from school that oxidation means basically, to rust, and that 'anti' means 'against' but in order to understand the role of antioxidants you need to understand what these agents are opposing. In much the same way as oxidation creates rust, causing a breakdown on the surface of inanimate objects, oxidation inside the body causes a breakdown of the cells. The particles produced by this breakdown are called free radicals and they attack healthy cells. This chain of of events weakens your immune functions and speeds up aging and studies show links to various forms of diseases, such as cancer, heart disease and many other degenerative conditions.

When you cut an apple or an avocado and squeeze lemon over the fruit, it will not go brown — or oxidise — but rather stay its original colour as you are preventing the process of oxidation, or at least slowing it down. The vitamin C, an antioxidant vitamin in the lemon, is doing it right in front of your eyes.

Ideally, we want to get rid of those 'radicals' and one way of doing this is to eat properly, avoid stress and cut back on the habits that promote them, such as smoking, drinking, eating poorly and the one we can't always avoid, pollution from the environment.

In basic terms, vegetables and fruits with the strongest colours are generally rich with antioxidants and high in vitamins and minerals. Oranges, red capsicums (peppers), tomatoes, spinach and carrots are all good examples of foods rich in these nutrients, to name a few. Culinary herbs and spices are also wonderful sources of powerful antioxidants and even when you add just a handful of fresh herbs to a salad you increase the antioxidant capacity of that salad by 200 per cent.

the good, the bad and the spooky

Every time I go to the doctor she checks my cholesterol levels — and for good reason. I know that smoking (luckily I don't smoke) and consuming foods high in fat (bad fat anyway) can push your cholesterol over the top. Interestingly, cholesterol only comes from animals and animal products — never from plants — so a diet rich in vegetables and fruits is looking better and better as I get older!

Although most of us think of it as a bad thing, cholesterol has a number of important functions in the body including the production of hormones, vitamin D and bile acids. A waxy substance, the majority of cholesterol in the body is made in the liver from saturated fats and the remainder comes from cholesterol in food.

Because cholesterol is a fatty substance, it doesn't dissolve in the bloodstream and needs to be transported around the body on a protein carrier called lipoprotein. The two major carriers of cholesterol are high-density lipoproteins (HDL), also know as 'good' cholesterol because they tend to take the cholesterol away from the arteries, back to the liver, and low-density lipoproteins (LDL), known as 'bad' cholesterol. I have come up with my own acronym to explain these: Happy and Delightful for the good fats and Lazy and Disgusting, for the fats we don't want!

It worries me when people try to take fats completely out of their diets to lose weight because we need some fats in our body to produce hormones and repair our cell membranes and for the creation of Vitamin D, for healthy bones and teeth. But if there is an excess of the LDL (the lazy bad dude) in our body, it ends up sticking to our arteries and causing all kinds of problems — they call it plaque. When this plaque builds up in the arteries of the heart and brain it can cause strokes and heart attacks.

The spooky part is that there are not necessarily any symptoms. This is why a healthy diet and exercise is so important. We need to keep the blood pumping to exercise the heart muscle, ensure our arteries are elastic, and keep an eye on our Happy and Lazy ratio.

The aim is to try and eat less saturated and

trans fats (both of which increase LDL cholesterol) and replace them with healthy fats, such as monounsaturated and polyunsaturated fats.

Over-consuming foods with saturated fats and trans fats in them can increase the risk of heart disease. These include foods like full-fat milk, cheese, butter and fatty meat products. Trans fats are unhealthy substances that are formed when oils are solidified during a chemical process called hydrogenation. Trans fats can also be found in things like take-away meals, packaged snacks, commercially packaged baked items such as crackers, biscuits, doughnuts, muffins, cakes, pies and processed meat products. These are all examples of foods that can contain fats that are not good for you. I admit that I do eat some of these foods (I'm human after all!) but in moderation — that is the key.

So what about the good fats? In general, monounsaturated and polyunsaturated fats can help lower blood cholesterol levels. Foods high in these fats include most nuts and seeds and a variety of vegetable oils. The two types of polyunsaturated fats that affect our health most positively are omega-3 and omega-6. According to the Australian Heart Foundation these can be found in oily fish, such as tuna, salmon, sardines and blue mackarel along with things like tahini, linseeds, sunflower and safflower oil, pine nuts, walnuts and brazil nuts.

I believe the most important of all these happy fats is omega-3. If you can't get it from fresh fish it can be obtained from good-quality fish oil supplements, flaxseed oil or oil derived from algae. As well as aiding with heart health by lowering blood pressure, blood fats and reducing the stickiness of platelets, omega-3s are also crucial for brain development and cognitive function and evidence has shown them to have anti-inflammatory effects. We should be trying to eat oily fish at least twice a week. All this and I find it also helps improve my hair and skin, too!

water, water all around and not a drop to drink

Wonderful refreshing and delicious, bubbly or flat, mineralised or distilled, PH balanced and alkaline — so many kinds of water!

I always love going to Australia, but especially because you can still fill a kettle for your cuppa with tap water. These days, in many parts of the world, it is considered a rarity to be able to do this.

It is commonly believed that between 60 and 70 per cent of our body is made up of water. The jury is out on exactly how much water we should consume daily, but it seems logical that we should at least replace what we lose every day in perspiration, elimination and breathing!

According to the Mayo Clinic based in the United States, we lose an average of about 1.5 litres (52 fl oz/6 cups) of fluid a day through perspiration and breathing, and another 1 litre (35 fl oz/ 4 cups) for elimination. By that maths, we need to drink at least 2.5 litres (87 fl oz/10 cups) of water to make up for all our bodily functions and help cleanse our system of toxins. I try to drink at least 1.5–2 litres (6–8 cups) water a day, including a coffee and a few cups of tea. Foods with a high water content, like most fruit and vegetables, can also count towards our fluid intake.

I notice throughout the day that I become very tired when I am dehydrated. I find that I will experience an afternoon lull when I have forgotten to drink water — and it often mimics hunger — an unfortunate mimic because it leads to snacking on all kinds of yummy bad food!

taking your pulses!

Our bodies need protein to repair cells. Meats and fish are probably the most well-known sources of protein, but protein can also be obtained from plants although most plant foods except soy do not supply all of the amino acids and so are often referred to as incomplete proteins. Good plant sources include a variety of legumes (when dried they are known as pulses) such as lentils and chickpeas; a variety of beans including red kidney, lima, pinto, black, white, butte, borlotti, haricot, cannellini, navy and adzuki beans; as well as split peas, nuts and seeds. Ideally, these should be combined with grains such as rice to make a 'complete protein'. Fermented soy products such as tempeh, miso and tofu are all complete proteins. Protein can also be found in some vegetables, including mushrooms, coconut, corn, peas, spirulina, algae and barley greens.

Eggs are also an excellent source of protein and choline, plus an array of minerals and other nutrients. We love them in our house and eat them almost every day!

It is true that eggs contain cholesterol but dietary cholesterol has very little bearing on blood cholesterol and it is generally believed that if you cut back on saturated and trans fats you should still be able to eat one egg a day without raising your cholesterol. I try to look for organic free-range eggs where the hens have been raised with freedom and without hormones and antibiotics. Happy hens make better eggs!

introduction

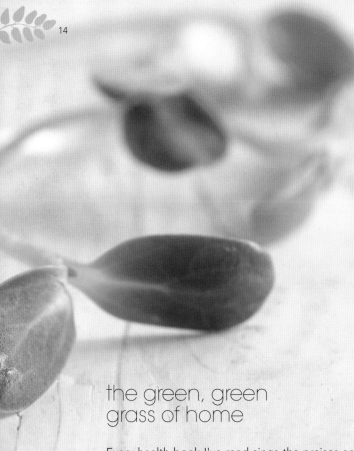

energy to all the cells in the body. They have anti-aging benefits and are recognised for their high level of enzyme activity. The most essential enzymes in sprouts are amylase, protease and lipase, which are all extremely helpful in aiding digestion.

sprouting can be fun

Good-quality sprouts are often available at health food stores, but you can also grow them yourself. The following seeds, grains and legumes can be sprouted. Only use organic seeds, legumes, grains and nuts for sprouting. Non-organic produce contains chemicals and may not sprout.

Seeds: alfalfa, broccoli, celery, clover, oats, radish, fenugreek, pepitas (pumpkin seeds), sunflower seeds.
Grains: buckwheat, barley, millet, rice, wheat.
Legumes: chickpeas, lentils, mung beans and soya beans.
Nuts: almonds, cashews, Hunza walnuts, pecans, pistachios.

Anyone, anywhere can create their own sprouts. All you need is the right equipment. You can either buy a ready-made kit that includes seeds, or alternatively you can create your own using 2 litre (70 fl oz/8 cup) capacity glass jars with a wide mouth. If you are using your own equipment you will also need a square of fly-screen gauze or some muslin (cheesecloth) that can be cut to size and used for lids, as well as a few rubber bands to fix the lid to the jar.

how to sprout

Place 2–4 tablespoons of any of the seeds or grains listed above in a jar — do not mix varieties as they will reach maturity at different times.

the green, green grass of home

Every health book I've read sings the praises and stresses the importance of green food and drinks in our diet. Near our home in Florida is an amazing place called the Hippocrates Health Institute. They are famous for their natural healthcare and were the first to introduce me to the value of wheatgrass. They grow it on the premises and juice it fresh several times daily. Within only a couple of days of drinking this nutritious, cleansing and 'living' drink I felt wonderfully alive and vital. The woman who founded Hippocrates, Ann Wigmore, claimed to have cured herself of cancer by eating 'live' foods (www.hippocratesinst.org). It's amazing to think that some of the world's largest and strongest creatures survive on grass alone. Not that I recommend that for us!

Sprouts are a living food that release and supply

14

Livwise

Pour in enough filtered pure water to half-fill the jar. Place the gauze over the top and seal with a rubber band. Leave to soak for at least 6 hours. Drain the seeds, rinse well and turn the jar upside down to drain completely — this prevents rotting.

Rinse with pure filtered water twice a day.

Germination will take place and the seeds and grains will expand by about eight times their original size (keep this in mind when adding them to the jar).

Legumes and nuts will not expand at the same rate as seeds and grains. Place 1 cup of legumes or nuts in a jar as above and fill with filtered pure water. Set aside at room temperature to soak for at least 15 hours. Continue to wash and drain the legumes and nuts twice a day, even after germination begins, until they are ready to eat. See the chart below for more details.

sweets for my sweet, sugar for my honey

As I said, I have a very sweet tooth but I try to steer clear of refined sugars. Instead, I use honey, maple syrup and the less well-known agave syrup, which has a lower glycemic index (GI) than sugar and is derived from the agave plant. It is available from most health food stores.

I also sometimes use a sugar substitute called xylitol, which is a natural sweetener, occurring in many fruits, vegetables and hardwoods, such as Birch, and tastes just like sugar. Xylitol has a very low GI and helps stabilise blood sugar and insulin levels. All in all, in small amounts, xylitol is a great sugar substitute for those with a sweet tooth.

Other sugar alternatives include the extracts from the stevia leaf, which are over 100 times

sprouting chart

TYPE	DRY MEASURE	READY TO EAT	YIELDS
Almonds	1 cup	2 days	2 cups
Alfalfa Seeds	3 tablespoons	4–5 days	4 cups
Sunflower Seeds	2 cups	1–2 days	2½ cups
Sesame Seeds	1 cup	1–2 days	1½ cups
Lentils	1 cup	3 days	4 cups
Mung Beans	½ cup	2–3 days	4 cups
Chickpea	1 cup	3 days	4 cups
Hulled Buckwheat	1 cup	1 day	2 cups
Wheat	1 cup	1 day	3 cups
Wild Rice	1 cup	1 day	3 cups

sweeter than sugar, if you can believe it is possible! It has been used in Peru and Brazil for many years to regulate blood sugar and aid digestion.

My new favourite, coconut palm sugar, is also a wonderful alternative to sugar and can be used as a substitute in any recipe calling for soft or dark brown sugar. It contains some B vitamins, potassium, magnesium, zinc and iron.

extra daily support

My husband John, is an incredibly wonderful and intelligent man, who has owned and run his dietary supplement business, Amazon Herb Company, for twenty years. He started out life as a treasure hunter and spent years searching the Amazon rainforest for treasures and ancient artifacts.

During his years of exploration in the rainforest, the indigenous people introduced him to the traditional use of therapeutic plants. After a health crisis and healing experience using botanicals, he realised a simple truth: the real treasure of the rainforest is, in fact, the life-enhancing properties of the rainforest plants. Now he is not only devoted to expanding the awareness of this healing potential but also protecting the precious resources of the Amazon for future generations.

The Amazon rainforest is an amazing place and its bountiful gifts to the world include fruits like avocados, coconuts, figs, oranges, lemons, grapefruit, bananas, guavas, pineapples, mangoes, tomatoes; vegetables including corn, potatoes, rice, pumpkin (winter squash) and yams; spices such as black and cayenne pepper, cocoa, cinnamon, cloves, ginger, sugar cane, turmeric, coffee, vanilla and some nuts, including Brazil nuts and cashews. At least 3000 fruits are found in the rainforests; of these only 200 are now in use in the Western world. The Indians of the rainforest use over 2000 of them. One of the greatest treasures that John has discovered (apart from me of course — ha ha!) is an amazing fruit known as camu camu.

Camu camu (*Myrciaria dubia*) grows naturally in the Amazon rainforest basin — it spends part of its life in the rainy season submerged in the

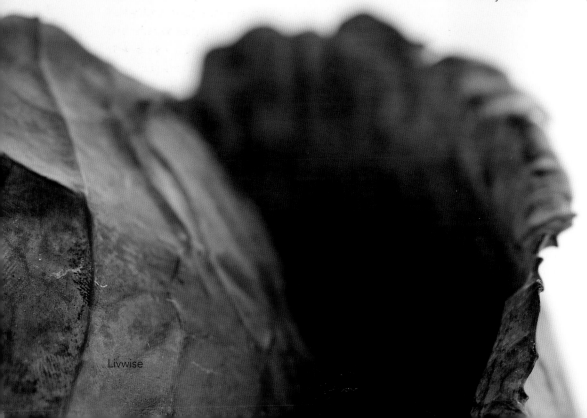

Amazon River soaking up all the nutrients of the rainforest. It is quickly gaining recognition as having the highest naturally-occurring concentration of vitamin C on the planet, beating out second-place acerola and having over thirty times the amount of vitamin C as an orange. It also contains amino acids, terpines, fibre, betacarotene, calcium, potassium, phosphorus, iron, and other beneficial substances. A recent study in Japan confirmed that camu camu is an antioxidant and also helps with inflammation.

The wonder of the rainforest, apart from its beauty and the abundance of life, is that there is so much to still be discovered. Only three per cent of the 100,000 plant species within the Amazon rainforest have been studied for their therapeutic value — and from this tiny percentage come the basis of about 25 per cent of our pharmaceuticals.

Along with a balanced diet I take a few vitamin supplements that I can't always get through food. Most of the time I try to take a multi-vitamin and mineral supplement, as well as a CQ10, Omega-3 and B-complex vitamin. In addition to these, I take Digestazon, Fiberzon, Camu Gold and many other Amazon Herb dietary supplements that help to aid my health and digestion. For more information go to www.amazonherb.net

let's get physical

It's funny really, that one of my most popular songs from the eighties is 'Let's get physical'. It's perfect for me because I've always loved exercise. I never find it a chore — I love to get up, get out and move my body. Every day I do some kind of activity, even if it is just walking my dog. I play tennis or go for a run around the block or use the treadmill, or I do yoga. I have to do something to expend energy or

I don't feel good. I even carry a skipping rope in my carry-on bag when I travel. Skipping stimulates the lymphatic system and helps strengthen your bones and heart, and it makes you feel young too! At Gaia we encourage our guests to walk, especially after meals — I feel best when in nature and in times of stress just getting outside and walking is a naturally healing thing for me to do.

everything in moderation

For me, the best way to stay healthy and trim is to eat what I like in moderation. I eat a little bit of everything so I'm not denying myself the pleasure of new flavours and experiences — I just don't eat it all! I find that the first few bites of dessert are amazing, but after a couple of mouthfuls the taste just isn't as exciting. That's the time to stop. You need to have willpower to continually make this decision. The easiest way I've found to eat less is to share my dessert with someone else, usually my husband, and it's more fun as well!

Your mind is very powerful in all aspects of health and to enjoy your food and appreciate where it comes from means your body will accept it with gratitude. My husband John and I travel a great deal and much of our lives are spent in hotels and on planes. We have learned to eat wisely and include as much fresh 'alive' food as we can. We never eat without giving thanks for the meal before us and taking a few silent moments to appreciate the miracle of the food before us, and all those who grew and prepared it. This expression of gratitude brings us into the moment and we enjoy our meal with the acknowledgement of all the energy and love that has gone into it, including the soil, the sun and the rain on our beautiful earth that made it all possible. Enjoy!

LivWise shopping list

* **lettuce** — a selection of salad leaves, bright, light and dark.
* **carrots**
* **celery**
* **tomatoes** — try to buy a variety of heirloom and cherry to use in different dishes.
* **onions** — I usually buy a variety of spring onions (scallions) and red onions.
* **beetroot** with the beetroot greens intact (which are great to serve, steamed, with eggs)
* **broccoli/kale/spinach/bok choy (pak choy)** — any or all of these can be added to a dish or steamed to make a wonderful side dish.
* **asparagus**
* **pumpkin (winter squash) and sweet potato**
* **lemons** — buy lots of these!
* **bananas**
* **blueberries**
* **raspberries**
* **cranberries, cherries and rhubarb in season**
* **almonds**
* **oatmeal and quinoa**
* **soy milk and organic low-fat dairy milk**
* **non-fat yoghurt**
* **honey** — I try to use this instead of sugar in tea. It can also help with allergies if you buy honey that is locally made from local hives.

* **maple syrup**
* **whole rye, pumpernickel or sourdough bread and crackers**
* **coconut palm sugar** (see page 15) my favourite sugar substitute!
* **olive oil and ghee**
* **sea salt and organic black pepper**
* **garlic**
* **olives**
* **Bragg Liquid Aminos** (see page 101)
* **cheese** — we love it and we eat small amounts of cheddar and love soft goat's cheese and brie.
* **butter** — love it! I have tried margarines and soy spreads over the years but I'm now back to the real thing!
* **pickled okra, dill cucumbers or capsicums** — pickled or fermented foods are good for digestion.
* **coconut water** — pure and delicious!
* **english breakfast tea or green tea**
* **coffee** — organic and as locally grown as possible.
* **fish** — especially salmon and preferably locally caught from sustainable sources.
* **organic free-range chicken and eggs**
* **a bar of dark chocolate at the check-out!**

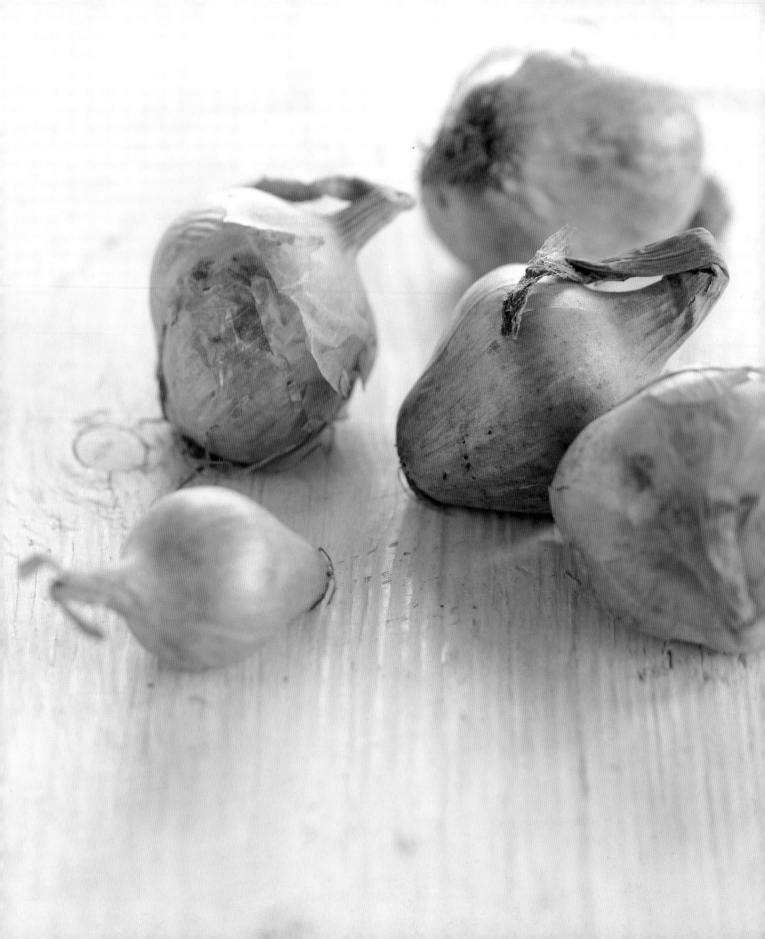

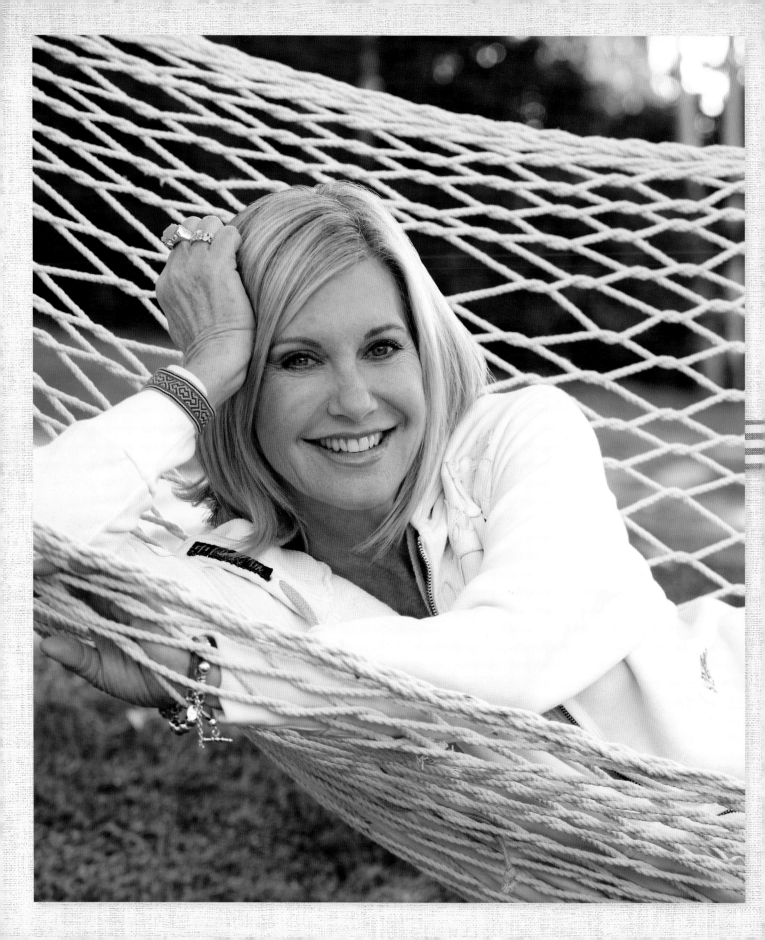

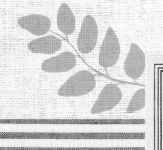

breakfast

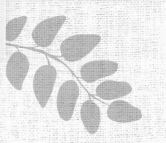

gaia toasted muesli
serves 8

400 g (14 oz/4 cups) rolled
   (porridge) oats
280 g (10 oz/2 cups) mixed raw,
   unsalted nuts and seeds,
   such as pecans, macadamia nuts
   or pepitas (pumpkin seeds)
60 g (2¼ oz/1 cup) shredded
   coconut
125 ml (4 fl oz/½ cup) macadamia
   oil
175 g (6 oz/½ cup) honey or raw
   agave syrup (see note)
pinch sea salt
125 g (4½ oz/1 cup) mixed
   currants, raisins and dried
   cranberries

Preheat the oven to 190°C (375°F/Gas 5). Line a large baking tray with baking paper.

Place the oats, nuts and seeds, coconut, macadamia oil, honey and salt in a large bowl and toss well to combine. Spread on the prepared baking tray and cook for about 25–30 minutes, stirring occasionally, until golden brown. Remove from the oven and allow to cool completely.

Toss the currants, cranberries and raisins through the oat mixture. Serve in bowls with milk, yoghurt and fresh seasonal fruit, if desired.

Toasted muesli can be stored in an airtight container for up to 2 weeks.

Note: Raw certified organic agave syrup is a concentrated fruit juice used as a sweetener that is commercially produced from several species of the agave plant. Be careful of the brands you buy — try and get certified organic agave syrup. It is available from most health food stores.

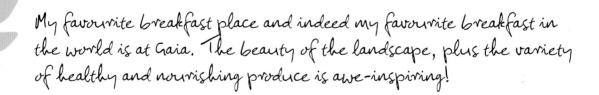

My favourite breakfast place and indeed my favourite breakfast in the world is at Gaia. The beauty of the landscape, plus the variety of healthy and nourishing produce is awe-inspiring!

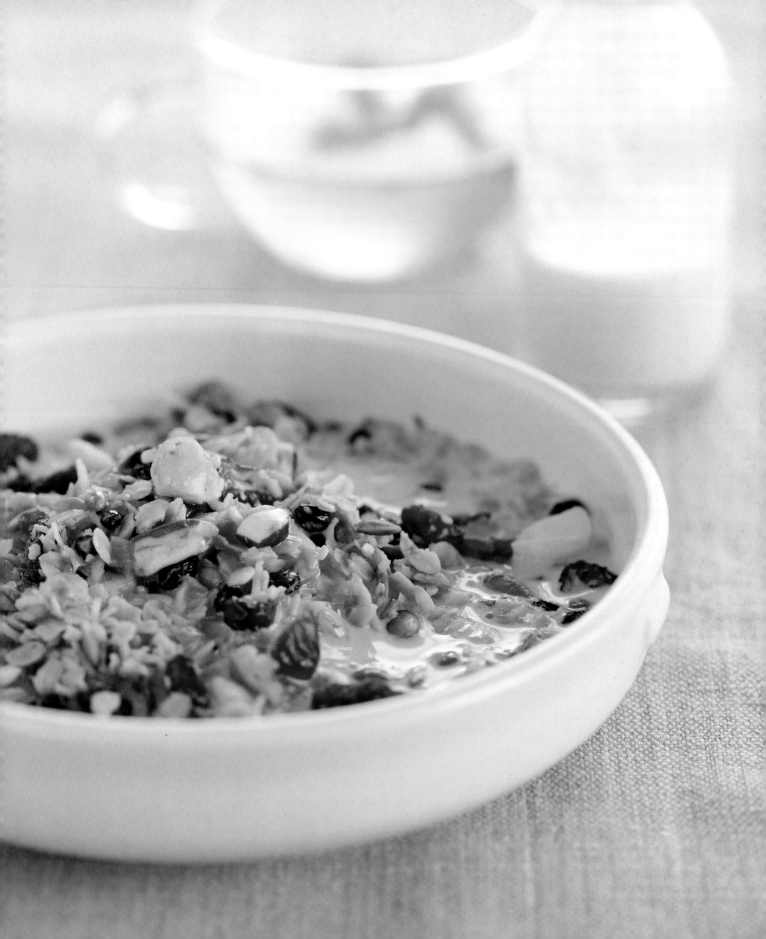

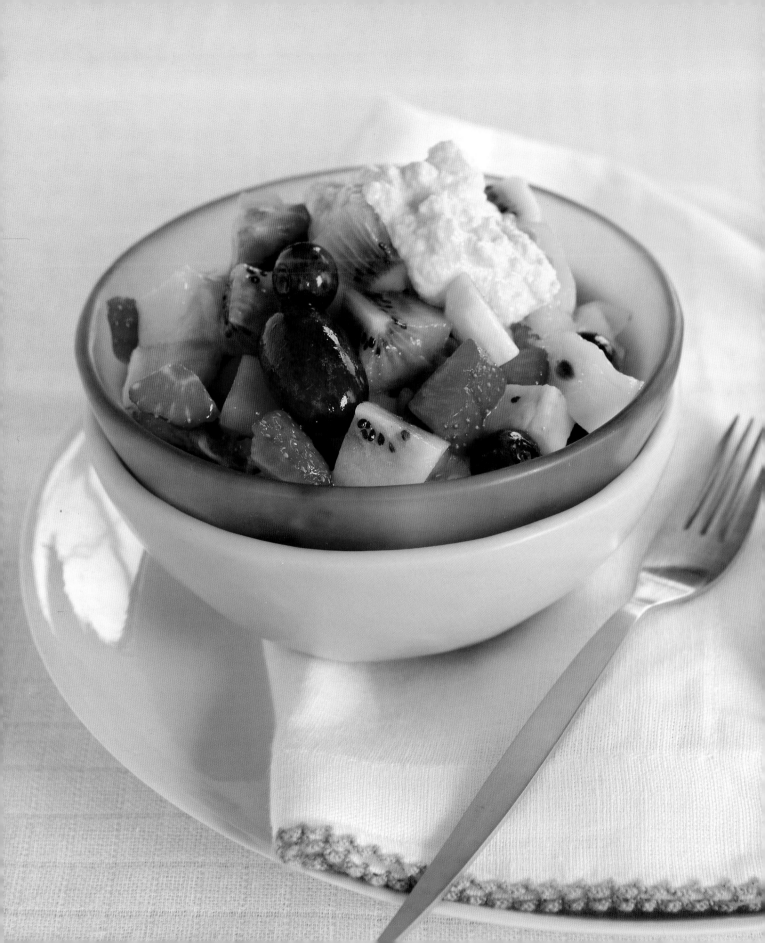

fruit salad with nut cream
serves 2

1 small banana, chopped
6 large strawberries, hulled and
    chopped
40 g (1½ oz/¼ cup) blueberries
2 kiwi fruit, chopped
185 g (6½ oz/1 cup) chopped red
    papaya
1 small mango, diced
90 g (3¼ oz/½ cup) seedless red
    or green grapes
2 passionfruit, pulp removed

NUT CREAM
80 g (2¾ oz/½ cup) unsalted raw
    cashews or almonds
60 ml (2 fl oz/¼ cup) non-dairy
    milk, such as oat, almond, rice
    or coconut milk

To make the nut cream, put the cashews in a small bowl and pour over 60 ml (2 fl oz/¼ cup) water. Cover with plastic wrap and refrigerate for at least 1 hour or overnight. Drain the nuts.

Put the nuts and milk in a food processor and process until well combined and smooth. Transfer to a bowl, cover and refrigerate until required.

To make the fruit salad, put the banana, strawberries, blueberries, kiwi fruit, papaya, mango, grapes and passionfruit pulp into a serving bowl and toss gently to combine. Serve the fruit salad with a dollop of the chilled nut cream on top.

Any leftover nut cream can be stored in an airtight container in the refrigerator for 1 day.

Note: When you are making the nut cream you can replace 40 g (1½ oz/¼ cup) of the nuts with macadamia nuts. You can also add a few drops of natural vanilla extract to the milk if you prefer a slightly sweeter flavour.

natural muesli
serves 8

200 g (7 oz/2 cups) organic rolled
  (porridge) oats
35 g (1¼ oz/¼ cup) organic
  oat bran
90 g (3¼ oz/1 cup) organic
  wheat germ
30 g (1 oz/¼ cup) organic pepitas
  (pumpkin seeds)
30 g (1 oz/¼ cup) organic
  sunflower seeds
30 g (1 oz/¼ cup) organic sultanas
  (golden raisins)
30 g (1 oz/¼ cup) organic raisins
35 g (1¼ oz/¼ cup) organic dried
  apricots, finely chopped
2 organic dried figs, finely
  chopped
15 g (½ oz/¼ cup) organic
  shredded coconut

Place the oats, oat bran, wheat germ, pepitas, sunflower seeds, sultanas, raisins, dried apricots and figs and coconut into a large bowl and toss well to combine. Add enough water just to cover the dry ingredients. Cover and refrigerate overnight.

Serve the muesli with non-dairy milk, yoghurt and fresh fruit, if desired.

Natural muesli can be stored in an airtight container for up to 2 weeks.

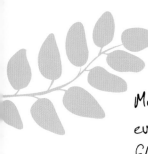

Muesli is one of my favourite breakfast dishes. My father had it every morning of his life. It provides nourishment, energy and fibre — what could be better than that?

bircher muesli with orange and yoghurt
serves 6

200 g (7 oz/2 cups) rolled
   (porridge) oats
125 ml (4 fl oz/½ cup) freshly
   squeezed orange juice
250 ml (9 fl oz/1 cup) yoghurt
   drink
250 g (9 oz/1 cup) plain yoghurt
2 tablespoons honey
125 g (4½ oz/1 cup) sultanas
   (golden raisins)
100 g (3½ oz) mixed fresh
   fruit, such as banana, apple,
   strawberries or kiwi fruit
60 g (2¼ oz/½ cup) slivered
   almonds, toasted

Put the oats, orange juice, yoghurt drink, yoghurt, honey and sultanas in a large bowl and stir well to combine. Cover with plastic wrap and refrigerate for at least 2 hours or overnight.

Just before serving, thinly slice or finely chop the fruit. Lightly fold the fruit and toasted slivered almonds through the oat mixture. Serve immediately.

Bircher muesli can be stored in an airtight container in the refrigerator for up to 1 day, but only add the fresh fruit just before serving.

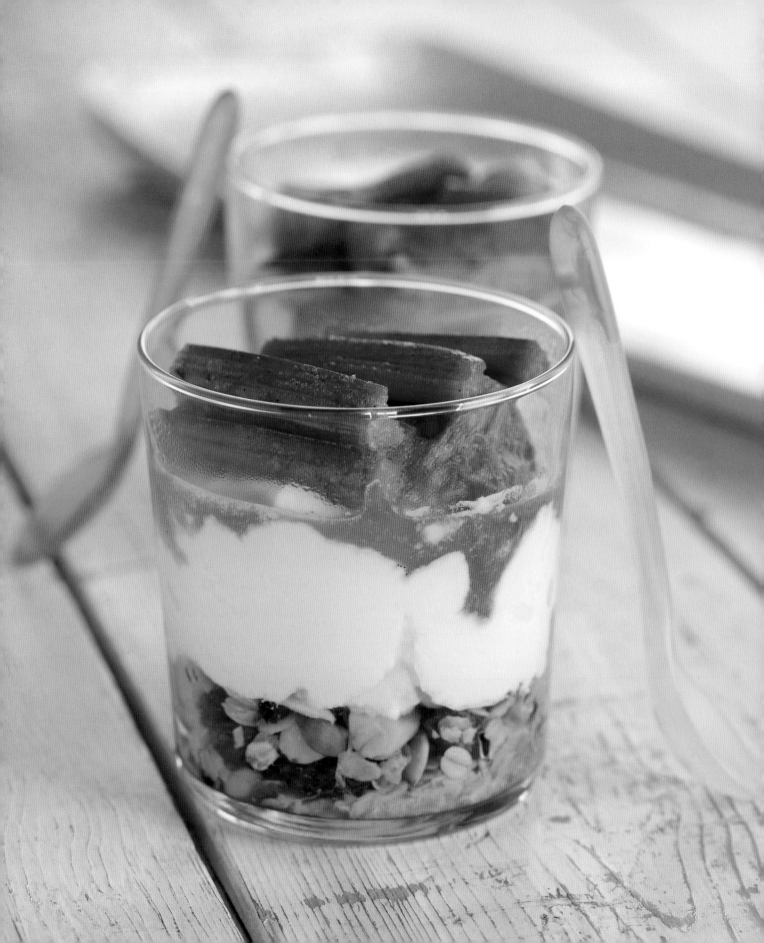

poached rhubarb
serves 6–8

750 g (1 lb 10 oz) rhubarb,
   trimmed and rinsed
1 vanilla bean, halved lengthways,
   seeds scraped
1 cinnamon stick
50 g (1¾ oz/¼ cup) light palm
   sugar (jaggery), roughly
   chopped
1 tablespoon apple juice
   concentrate
2 teaspoons natural vanilla extract
125 ml (4 fl oz/½ cup) freshly
   squeezed orange juice

Cut the rhubarb into 6 cm (2½ inch) lengths. Place the rhubarb into a large saucepan. Add the vanilla seeds and pod, cinnamon stick, palm sugar, apple concentrate, vanilla extract and orange juice. Add 125 ml (4 fl oz/½ cup) water. Bring to the boil over high heat, then reduce the heat to low and simmer for 5–10 minutes, or until the rhubarb is soft but still holding its shape. Remove from the heat and set aside to cool.

Serve the rhubarb with plain yoghurt and muesli.

Leftover rhubarb can be stored in an airtight container in the refrigerator for up to 4 days.

Ah rhubarb! This recipe is another Gaia staple that I adore. It conjures strong memories of my childhood, when my mother would cook different fruits so at any time I could open the fridge and find a tempting jar filled with delicious stewed fruit — yum!

poached eggs with coriander pesto
serves 2

pinch sea salt
4 free-range eggs
2 slices toasted sourdough bread,
   to serve

CORIANDER PESTO
(makes 1½ cups)
2 cups firmly packed fresh
   coriander (cilantro) leaves
170 ml (5½ fl oz/⅔ cup) extra
   virgin olive oil
4 garlic cloves, quartered
50 g (1¾ oz/⅓ cup) Brazil nuts
40 g (1½ oz/⅓ cup) sunflower
   seeds
50 g (1¾ oz/⅓ cup) pepitas
   (pumpkin seeds)
freshly squeezed juice of 1 lemon

To make the coriander pesto, place all the ingredients into a food processor and process to a smooth paste. Set aside. This pesto can be made ahead of time and stored in an airtight container in the refrigerator for at least 1 week. Pesto can also be frozen for up to 3 months.

Half-fill a large deep frying pan with water, add the salt and place over medium heat. Working with one egg at a time, crack the egg into a small cup. When the water is just simmering, use a large spoon to stir the water in one direction to create a whirlpool. Carefully slip the egg into the centre of the whirlpool and poach for 1–2 minutes for a soft-poached egg, or until cooked to your liking. Remove with a slotted spoon to a plate, set aside and keep warm. Repeat with the remaining eggs until all are cooked.

Serve the warm poached eggs on the toast with a dollop of coriander pesto on top.

Note: Fresh coriander is an excellent blood purifier; 2 teaspoons of coriander pesto every day for 3–4 weeks is known to remove heavy metals from the body. Heavy metals include mercury, lead and aluminium. This pesto also goes well with baked potatoes, pasta and rice.

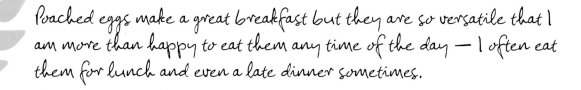

Poached eggs make a great breakfast but they are so versatile that I am more than happy to eat them any time of the day — I often eat them for lunch and even a late dinner sometimes.

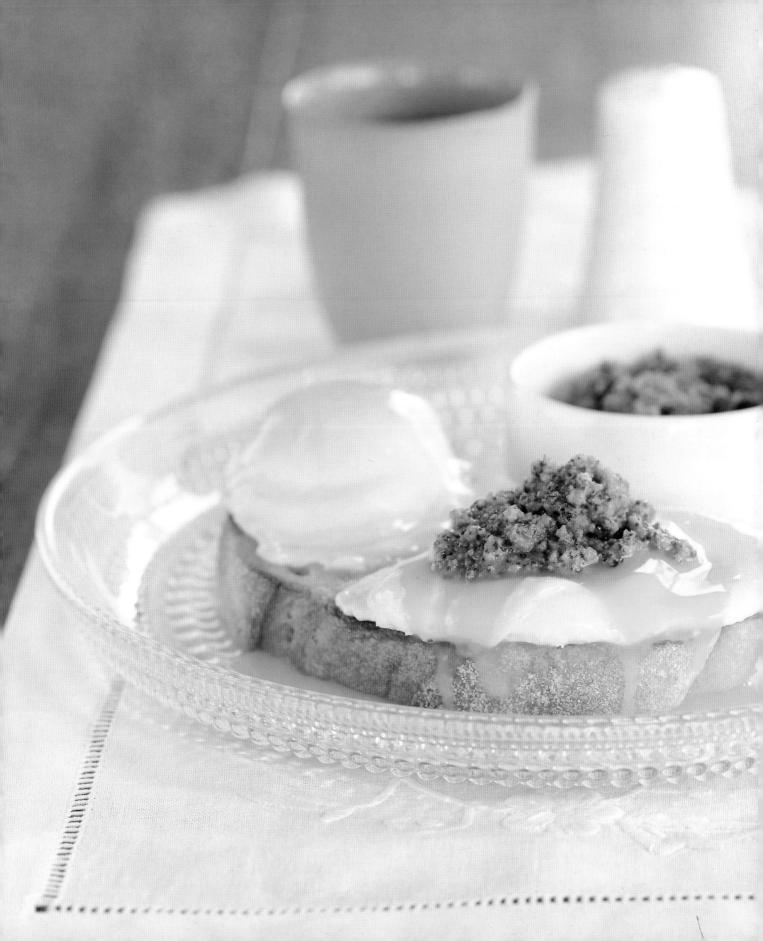

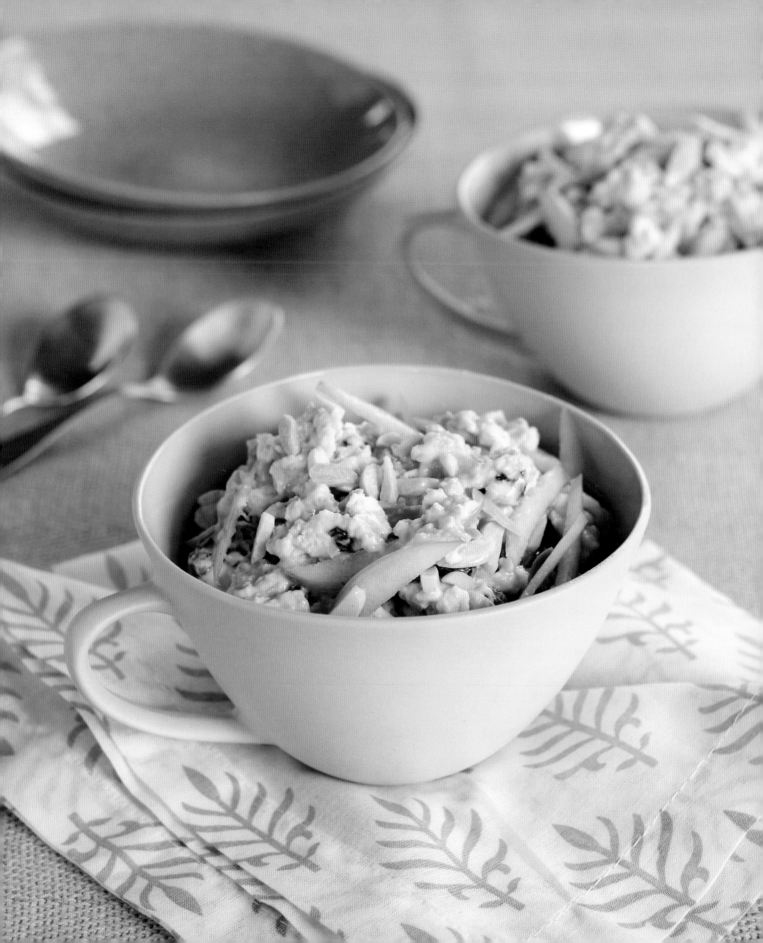

bircher muesli with apple and coconut
serves 2

100 g (3½ oz/1 cup) natural muesli (see page 26)

1 granny smith apple, peeled and coarsely grated, plus thin wedges of apple, extra, to serve (optional)

20 g (¾ oz/⅓ cup) shredded coconut

250 ml (9 fl oz/1 cup) non-dairy milk, such as oat, almond, rice or coconut milk

1 tablespoon xylitol (see note), plus extra, to serve (optional)

Put the muesli, grated apple, coconut, milk and xylitol in a bowl and stir well to combine. Cover with plastic wrap and refrigerate for at least 1 hour or overnight.

Divide the mixture between two serving bowls and serve with a little extra xylitol over the top for sweetness and the extra apple wedges if you like.

Note: Xylitol is a natural substance that is derived from fruit, vegetables and birch trees; it is also produced naturally in our bodies. Xylitol is a chemical-free, natural alternative to sugar and other artificial sweeteners. It is available from most health food stores.

protein and calcium-enriched muesli with fruit
serves 2

45 g (1¾ oz/⅓ cup) natural muesli
(see page 26)
non-dairy milk, such as oat,
almond, rice or coconut milk or
water
375 g (13 oz/2 cups) chopped
red papaya
2 kiwi fruit, chopped
12 strawberries, hulled and
halved
115 g (4 oz/¾ cup) blueberries
2 passionfruit, pulp removed
2 teaspoons bee pollen (see notes)
1 teaspoon maca powder
(optional) (see notes)
250 g (9 oz/1 cup) plain yoghurt
or 250 ml (9 fl oz/1 cup)
coconut milk

SEED AND NUT MIXTURE
1 tablespoon sunflower seeds
1 tablespoon linseeds
1 tablespoon pepitas (pumpkin
seeds)
2 teaspoons sesame seeds
2 teaspoons chopped blanched
almonds
2 teaspoons chopped Brazil nuts

To make the seed and nut mixture, use a spice grinder or coffee grinder to grind the seeds and nuts together until very finely chopped. Alternatively, soak all of the ingredients in just enough liquid to cover for at least 2 hours or overnight. Refrigerate until needed and drain before using.

Place the muesli and liquid of your choice in a bowl and stir well to combine. Cover with plastic wrap and refrigerate for at least 1 hour or overnight.

Put the papaya, kiwi fruit, strawberry, blueberries, passionfruit pulp, pollen, maca powder, if using, and yoghurt in a bowl. Add 2 tablespoons of the seed and nut mixture and the soaked muesli and stir gently to combine. Divide between serving bowls and serve immediately.

Notes: Bee pollen contains the richest known source of vitamins (particularly B vitamins) and minerals, enzymes to aid digestion, amino acids, hormones and fats. It is available from health food stores.

Maca (*Lepidium meyenii*) is an herbaceous plant native to Peru. Maca powder is rich in essential minerals, especially selenium, calcium, magnesium and iron, and includes fatty acids including linolenic acid, palmitic acid and oleic acids, as well as polysaccharides. Maca powder is believed to improve stamina, strength and energy, and is also a hormonal tonic. It can be added to water, juice, cereals, smoothies, juice, yoghurt or herbal teas. Take ½–2 teaspoons 6 days a week (have one day off). Like superfoods, such as barley grass, wheatgrass and bee pollen, maca helps to alkalise urine, thereby helping to mobilise toxins in the body. It is available from health food stores.

strawberry and macadamia bircher muesli
serves 2

250 g (9 oz) strawberries, hulled

100 g (3½ oz/1 cup) natural
   muesli (see page 26)

125 ml (4 fl oz/½ cup) non-dairy
   milk, such as oat, almond, rice
   or coconut milk

40 g (1½ oz/¼ cup) macadamia
   nuts, chopped, plus extra,
   to serve

1 tablespoon xylitol (see note
   page 33)

Cut 125 g (4½ oz) of the strawberries in half. Put the cut strawberries, muesli, milk, nuts and xylitol into a bowl and stir well to combine. Cover with plastic wrap and refrigerate for at least 1 hour or overnight.

Finely chop the remaining strawberries. Divide the muesli between serving bowls and serve with the diced strawberries and extra nuts scattered on top.

The basis of muesli is oats. If you have a gluten intolerance you can replace the oats with gluten-free corn flakes, buckwheat flakes or quinoa flakes.

almond pancakes with berries and yoghurt
serves 2

125 g (4½ oz) strawberries, hulled
   and quartered
80 g (2¾ oz/½ cup) blueberries
80 g (2¾ oz/⅔ cup) raspberries
1 tablespoon xylitol (see note
   page 33)
mint leaves, to serve
shredded coconut, to serve
90 g (3¼ oz/⅓ cup) plain yoghurt,
   to serve

ALMOND PANCAKES
70 g (2½ oz/⅔ cup) ground
   almonds
1 teaspoon bicarbonate of soda
   (baking soda)
2 tablespoons plain yoghurt
2 tablespoons xylitol (see note
   page 33)
2 free-range eggs, lightly beaten
2 teaspoons coconut oil (see note)

Combine all of the berries in a bowl. Purée one-quarter of the mixed berries with the xylitol in a food processor or blender until smooth. Set aside.

To make the pancakes, put the ground almonds, bicarbonate of soda, yoghurt, xylitol, egg and 1 tablespoon water in a mixing bowl and stir until a smooth batter forms, adding more water if needed.

Heat half of the coconut oil in a large frying pan over medium–high heat. Spoon half of the pancake mixture into the pan and cook for 2–3 minutes, or until bubbles appear on the surface. Carefully turn the pancake over and cook for a further 1–2 minutes, or until cooked through. Transfer to a heatproof serving plate and keep warm in a low oven. Repeat with the remaining oil and pancake batter to make 2 pancakes in total.

Serve the warm almond pancakes topped with mixed berries, berry purée, mint leaves and shredded coconut. Serve with yoghurt on the side.

Note: Coconut oil is available from health food stores and some grocery stores.

I love pancakes and when they are made with ground almonds, they make a healthy Sunday morning treat — the berries providing antioxidants and fibre with hardly any kilojoules. It doesn't get much better than that!

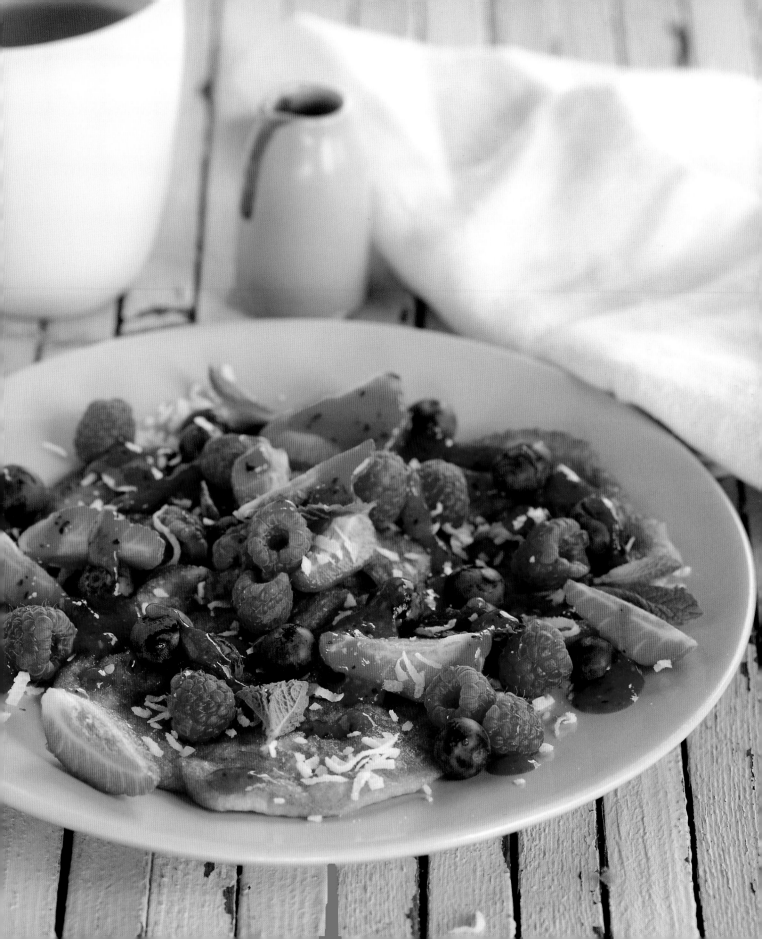

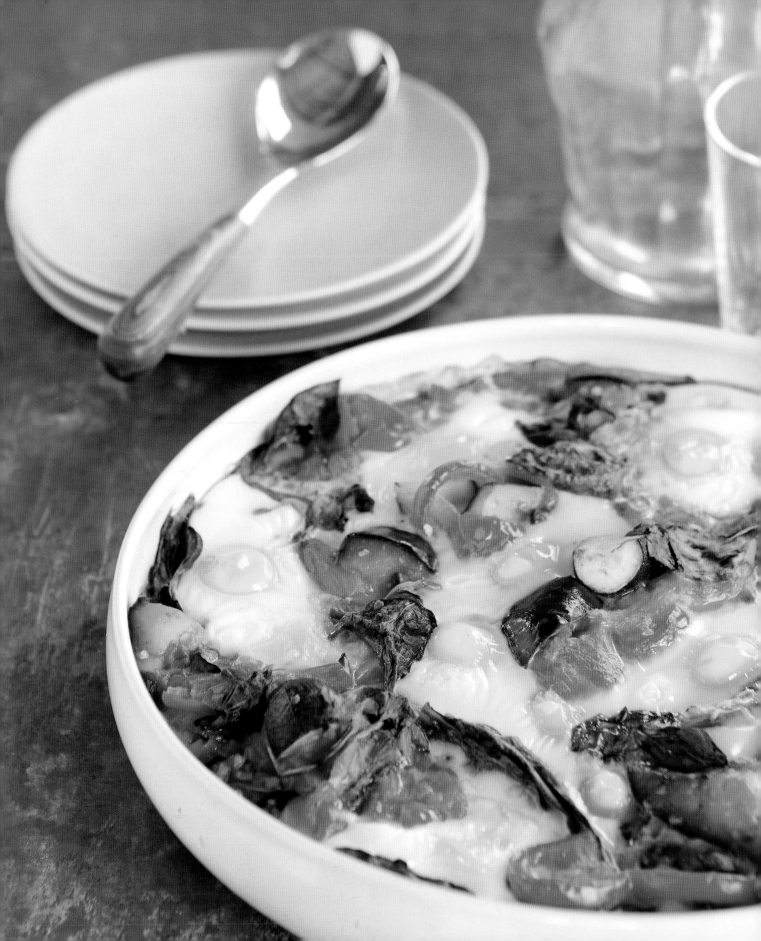

chakchouka baked eggs
serves 4

1 tablespoon olive oil

1 small brown onion, finely chopped

400 g (14 oz) tin whole tomatoes

250 g (9 oz/1²/₃ cups) cherry tomatoes, halved

1 tablespoon tomato paste (concentrated purée)

1 zucchini (courgette), chopped

½ red capsicum (pepper), seeded, membrane removed and thinly sliced

½ yellow capsicum (pepper), seeded, membrane removed and thinly sliced

½ small eggplant (aubergine), chopped

80 g (2¾ oz/1¾ cups) baby spinach leaves

8 free-range eggs

Preheat the oven to 200°C (400°F/Gas 6).

Heat the olive oil in a large saucepan over medium–high heat. Add the onion and cook for 5 minutes, or until softened. Add the tomatoes, cherry tomato and tomato paste and bring to the boil. Add the zucchini, capsicum and eggplant, then reduce the heat to medium–low and simmer for about 20 minutes, or until the vegetables are tender. Stir in the spinach. Transfer the vegetable mixture to a 1.5 litre (52 fl oz/6 cup) capacity ovenproof dish. Make eight indents in the mixture to fit the eggs.

Crack the eggs into the indents in the vegetable mixture. Bake in the oven for about 10–15 minutes, or until the eggs are just set. Serve immediately.

Tip: Traditionally, Chakchouka is made with leftover vegetables from the previous night's dinner. You can also serve the Chakchouka with fresh feta cheese crumbled over the top.

steamed egg custard with shiitake mushrooms and plain yoghurt

serves 4

olive oil spray, for cooking
2 fresh shiitake mushrooms, sliced
½ brown onion, chopped
4 free-range eggs
160 g (5¾ oz/⅔ cup) plain
  yoghurt
2 chives, snipped, to serve
4 slices toasted soy and linseed
  bread, cut into fingers, to serve

Heat a frying pan over medium–high heat. Spray the pan with the oil, add the mushroom and onion, and cook for 5 minutes, or until the onion has softened. Remove from the heat and set aside.

Whisk together the eggs and yoghurt, then season with salt and freshly ground black pepper. Stir through the mushroom and onion mixture.

Pour the egg mixture evenly among four 125 ml (4 fl oz/ ½ cup) capacity ramekins or ovenproof dishes. Place the ramekins in a bamboo steamer and cover with the lid. Fill a wok one-third full with water and bring to the boil over high heat. Place the steamer in the wok (making sure it doesn't touch the water) and steam for 8 minutes, or until the custards are just set.

Sprinkle the chives over the egg custards and serve with the toast fingers on the side.

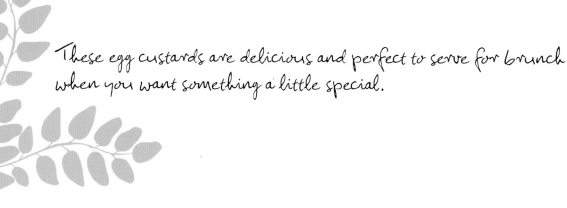

These egg custards are delicious and perfect to serve for brunch when you want something a little special.

ricotta fruit topping
makes 250 g (9 oz/1 cup)

45 g (1¾ oz/¼ cup) dried apricots
125 g (4½ oz/½ cup) fresh ricotta
  cheese
pinch ground cinnamon

Put the dried apricots in a bowl with 250 ml (9 fl oz/1 cup) water. Cover with plastic wrap and leave to soak overnight.

Drain the apricots, reserving the soaking liquid. Put the apricots and 125 ml (4 fl oz/½ cup) of the soaking liquid into a blender and blend until smooth. Add the ricotta cheese and cinnamon and blend until smooth. Transfer to a bowl and serve as an accompaniment to stewed, fresh or tinned fruit.

This ricotta fruit topping can be stored in an airtight container in the refrigerator for up to 2 days.

Tip: Instead of the soaked dried apricots you can try using unsweetened tinned peaches and a little of their juice; or homemade stewed apple puréed with a pinch of ground cloves and 1 teaspoon honey. Alternatively you can add soaked pitted prunes and their soaking juice; or add the finely grated zest and juice of 1 orange.

baked balsamic vegetables with ricotta

serves 4

olive oil spray, for cooking

2 tablespoons extra virgin olive
    oil

2 teaspoons balsamic vinegar

2 large roma (plum) tomatoes,
    halved

4 large mushrooms, trimmed

1 red onion, thinly sliced

1 small fennel bulb, trimmed, cut
    into 1 cm (½ inch) slices

2 garlic cloves, finely chopped

60 g (2¼ oz/¼ cup) crumbled
    fresh ricotta cheese

4 slices toasted sourdough bread,
    to serve

Preheat the oven to 180°C (350°F/Gas 4). Lightly grease a baking tray with the oil spray.

Whisk the olive oil and balsamic vinegar together in a small bowl until well combined.

Layer the tomato halves, mushrooms, onion, fennel, garlic and cheese on the prepared tray to create four small stacks. Drizzle with the oil mixture. Bake for 25 minutes, or until the vegetables have browned and are tender, and the cheese has melted slightly.

Serve each vegetable stack on a slice of the toasted sourdough bread.

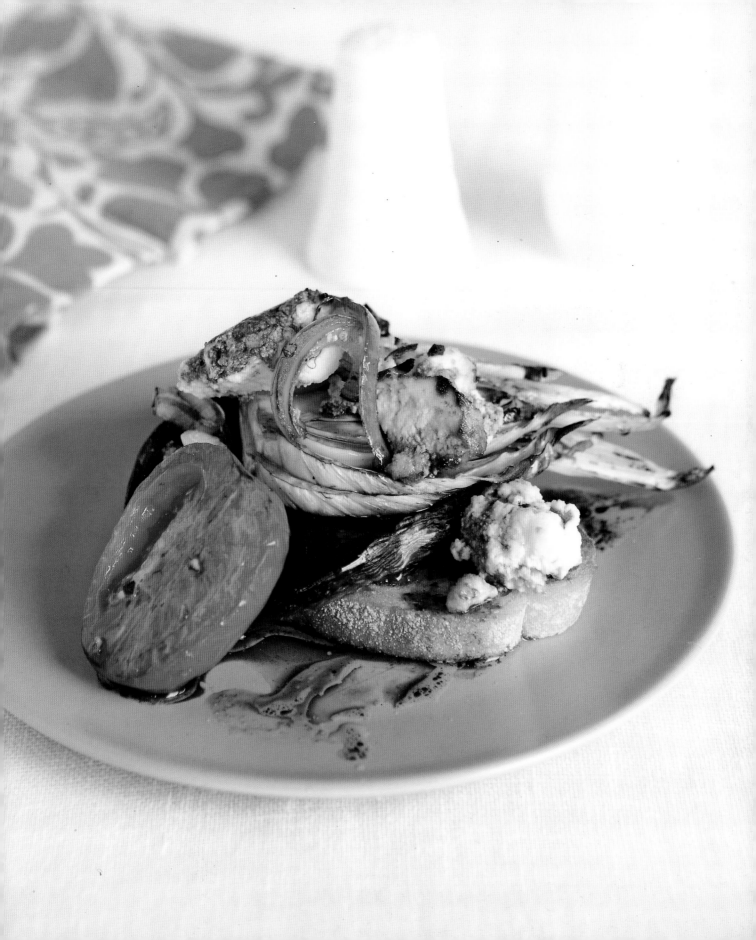

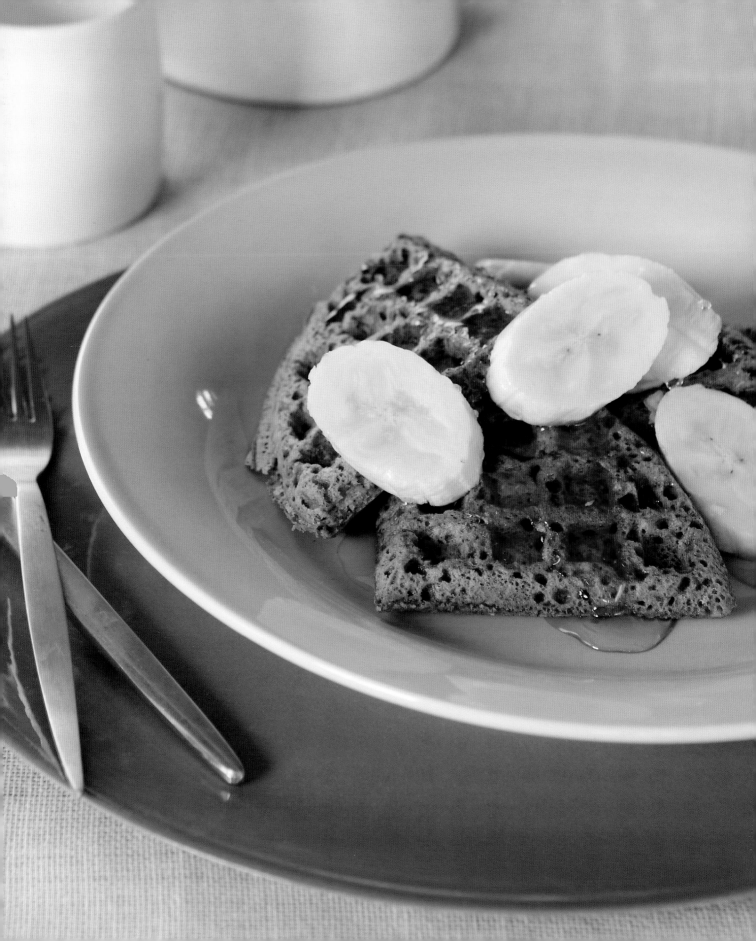

buckwheat waffles
serves 4

170 g (6 oz/1⅓ cups) buckwheat
  flour, sifted twice
95 g (3¼ oz/½ cup) cooked
  medium-grain brown rice
½ teaspoon sea salt
1 banana, sliced, to serve
honey, to serve

Put the flour and 185 ml (6 fl oz/¾ cup) water in a bowl and stir well to combine. Cover with plastic wrap and set aside for at least 1 hour.

Transfer the flour mixture to a blender and add the cooked rice, salt and 250 ml (9 fl oz/1 cup) hot water. Blend until well combined and smooth.

Heat a waffle maker following the manufacturer's instructions. Pour one-quarter of the batter mixture into the heated waffle maker and cook for 5 minutes, or until the waffle is golden and cooked through. Remove the waffle, transfer to a plate and keep warm. Repeat with the remaining batter to make four waffles in total.

Serve the warm waffles topped with the banana slices and a little honey.

Tip: You can wrap any leftover waffles in plastic wrap and freeze for up to 3 months. Warm the waffles straight from the freezer in a toaster or preheated oven before serving.

fresh herb omelettes with balsamic mushrooms

serves 2

1 tablespoon coconut oil (see
  note page 36) or ghee
125 g (4½ oz) button mushrooms,
  halved
1 tablespoon balsamic vinegar
6 free-range eggs
2 tablespoons finely chopped
  flat-leaf (Italian) parsley
2 tablespoons finely snipped
  chives
2 tablespoons finely chopped
  basil
2 tablespoons finely chopped
  thyme
mixed lettuce leaves, to serve

Heat half of the coconut oil in a frying pan over medium–high heat. Add the mushrooms and cook for about 5 minutes, stirring often, until cooked and golden brown. Remove from the heat and stir in the balsamic vinegar. Set aside and keep warm.

Put the eggs and 2 tablespoons water into a bowl and whisk until just combined. Add the herbs and mix well.

Heat 1 teaspoon of the remaining coconut oil in a frying pan over medium–high heat. Pour half of the egg mixture into the pan, swirling to coat the base. Cook for 1–2 minutes, or until almost set. Fold the omelette in half, remove to a serving plate and keep warm. Repeat with the remaining oil and egg mixture to make another omelette.

Serve the warm omelettes with the sautéed balsamic mushrooms and the lettuce leaves on the side.

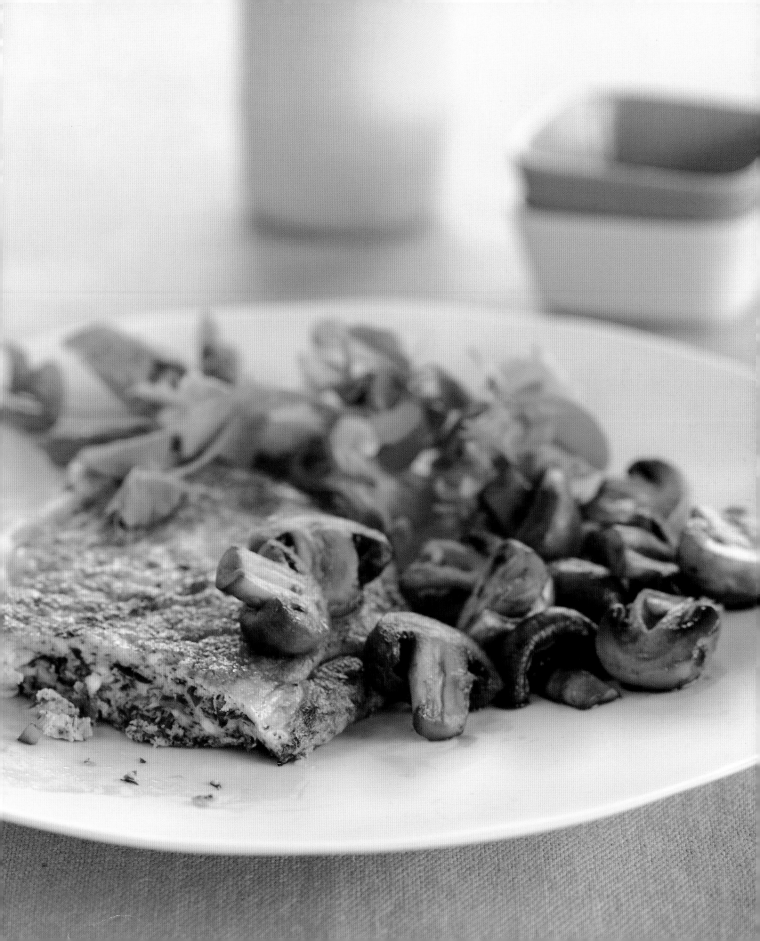

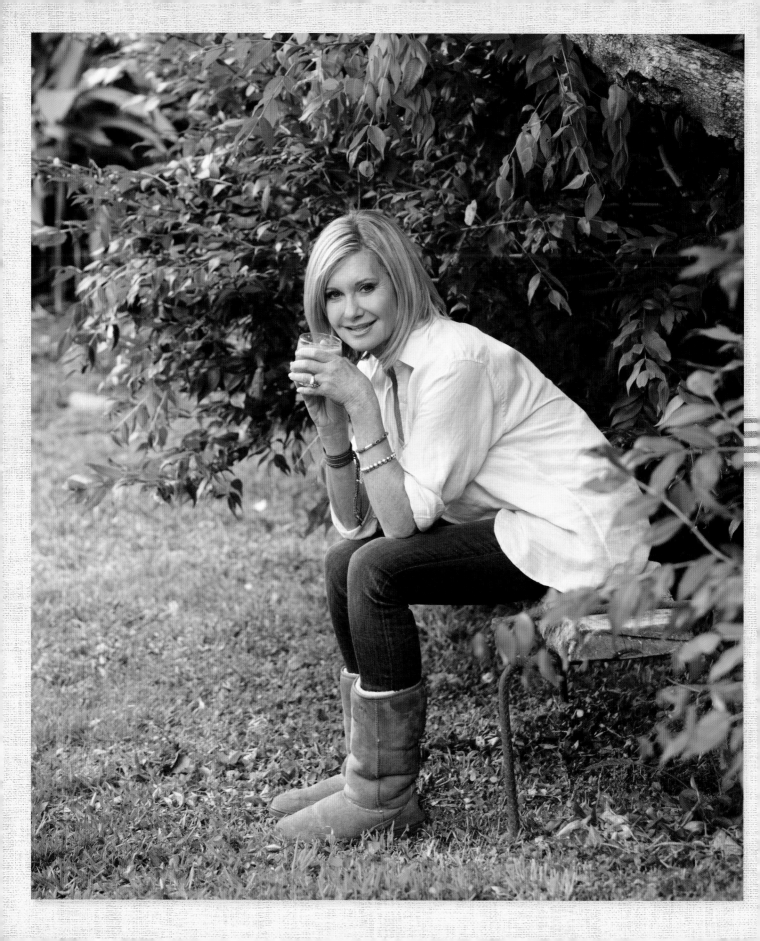

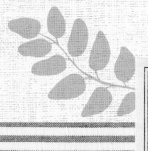

shakes, smoothies and juices

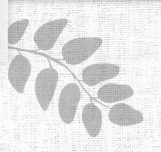

pina colada breakfast shake
serves 1

250 ml (9 fl oz/1 cup) fresh
   pineapple juice
250 ml (9 fl oz/1 cup) coconut
   milk
2 tablespoons coconut oil (see
   note page 36)
2 tablespoons protein powder
   (see note)
¼ cup ice cubes

Put all of the ingredients into a blender and blend until the ice is crushed and the mixture is smooth. Serve immediately.

Note: When selecting a protein powder make sure it is either raw or what is called undenatured protein powder, as this type of protein powder supports the immune system. It has the ability to detoxify the cells and support cellular repair and is a very digestible source of protein. Denatured products have been heated and this process means they lose certain immune-enhancing ingredients; many protein powders are also full of sugar. You can purchase good protein powders from most health food stores.

papaya and orange breakfast shake
serves 1

185 g (6½ oz/1 cup) chopped red
   papaya
freshly squeezed juice of 1 orange
250 ml (9 fl oz/1 cup) non-dairy
   milk, such as oat, almond, rice
   or coconut milk
¼ teaspoon natural vanilla extract
1 teaspoon green barley grass
   powder (see note)
1 teaspoon maca powder (see
   note page 34)

Put all of the ingredients into a blender and blend until well combined and smooth. Serve immediately.

Note: Green barley grass (*Hordeum vulgare*) powder comes from the seedling of the barley plant. It is usually harvested about 200 days after germination, when the shoots are less than 30 cm (12 inches). It is a concentrated source of nearly three dozen vitamins and minerals and is particularly rich in vitamins, calcium, iron, potassium and chlorophyll. Unlike most plants, barley grass provide all nine essential amino acids (those which your body can't produce). It is available in powdered form from most health food stores.

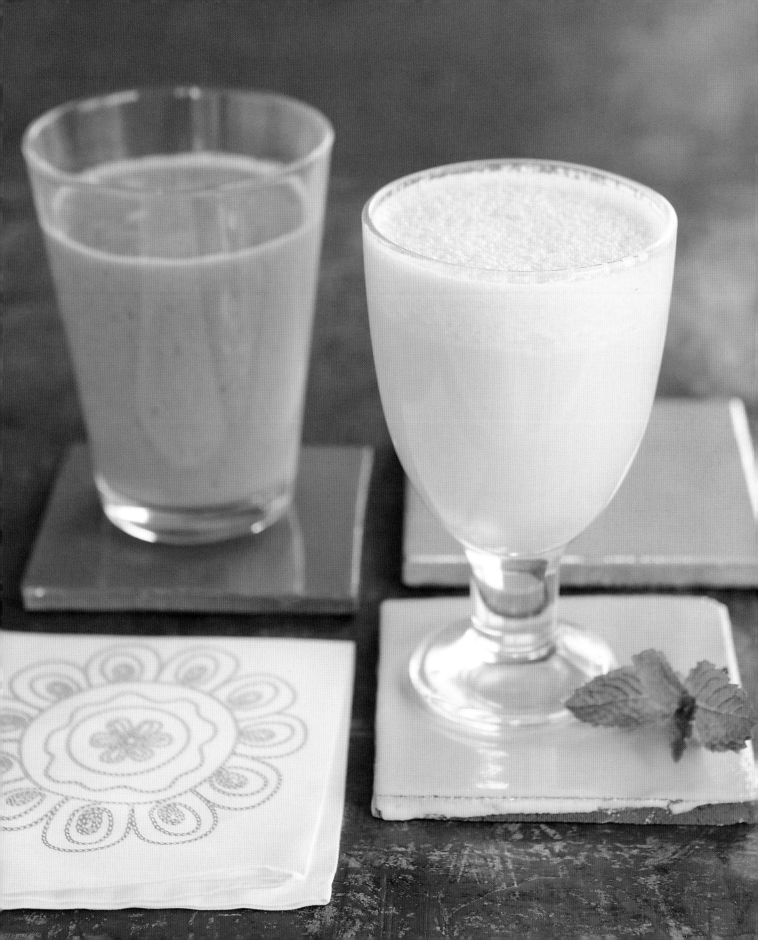

sprouted seed and pineapple smoothie
serves 1

½ cup sprouted alfalfa seeds
    (see pages 14–15)
2 tablespoons sprouted sesame
    seeds (see pages 14–15)
80 g (2¾ oz/½ cup) chopped
    pineapple
375 ml (13 fl oz/1½ cups) non-
    dairy milk, such as oat, almond,
    rice or coconut milk

Put all of the ingredients into a blender and blend until well combined and smooth. Serve immediately.

something-to-glow-about drink
serves 2

1 guava, peeled and coarsely
    chopped
1 kiwi fruit, peeled and coarsely
    chopped
125 ml (4 fl oz/½ cup) freshly
    squeezed orange juice
1 teaspoon freshly squeezed
    lime juice
1 passionfruit, pulp removed

Put the guava and kiwi fruit in a blender and blend until smooth. Add the orange and lime juices and blend again until well combined and smooth. Stir through the passionfruit pulp and serve immediately.

Note: Instead of kiwi fruit you can peel and dice ¼–½ pink grapefruit. For added tang add a little finely grated lime zest. Don't purée the passionfruit pulp as the seeds can release a bitter flavour, just stir it through.

almond milk
makes 375 ml (13 fl oz/1½ cups)

310 g (11 oz/2 cups) blanched almonds

Thoroughly rinse the almonds under cold running water, then place in a large bowl and cover with cold water. Set aside to soak for 12 hours. Rinse and drain well.

Put the almonds into a blender with 1.5 litres (52 fl oz/6 cups) cold water and blend until smooth — be careful not to blend the mixture for too long as it may become hot. Strain the milk through a square of muslin (cheesecloth). Serve chilled.

Almond milk can be stored in a sealed container in the refrigerator for up to 5 days.

Variations: You can use hazelnuts or Brazil nuts instead of the almonds. These varieties of nuts do not require soaking. You can also try adding 1 tablespoon linseeds (flaxseed) or honey to make a sweetened almond milk.

banana, pear and yoghurt smoothie
serves 1

1 small ripe pear, peeled, cored and chopped
1 banana, coarsely chopped
125 g (4½ oz/½ cup) plain yoghurt
125 ml (4 fl oz/½ cup) fresh apple juice

Put all of the ingredients into a blender and blend until well combined and smooth. Serve immediately.

sprouted wheat and fig smoothie

serves 1

3 dried figs, coarsely chopped
¼ cup sprouted wheat seeds
   (see page 14–15)
125 ml (4 fl oz/½ cup) almond
   milk (see page 53) or other
   non-dairy milk, such as oat, rice
   or coconut milk

Place the figs in a small bowl. Cover with water and set aside to soak for 30 minutes, or until softened. Drain well.

Put the drained softened figs, sprouted wheat seeds and almond milk in a blender with 125 ml (4 fl oz/½ cup) water and blend until well combined and smooth. Serve immediately.

apple, pear and guava juice

serves 2

2 granny smith apples, cored and
   quartered
2 pears, cored and quartered
2 guavas, peeled

Using an electric juice extractor, juice the apple, pear and guavas into a jug.

Pour into serving glasses and serve immediately.

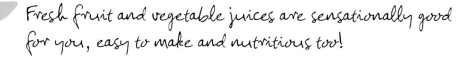

Fresh fruit and vegetable juices are sensationally good for you, easy to make and nutritious too!

Livwise

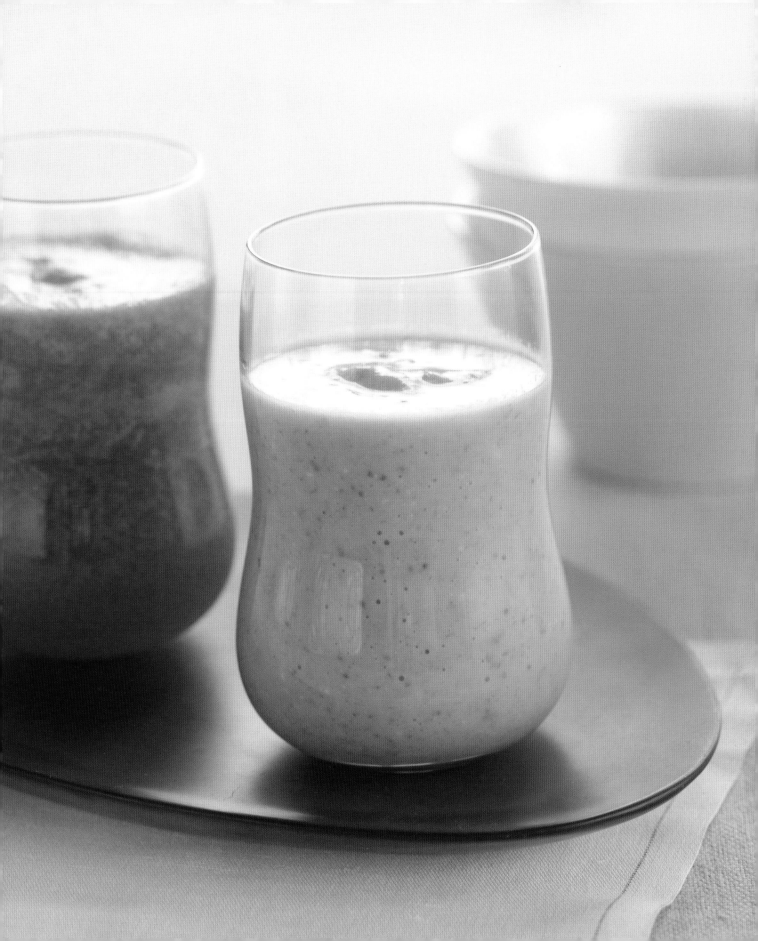

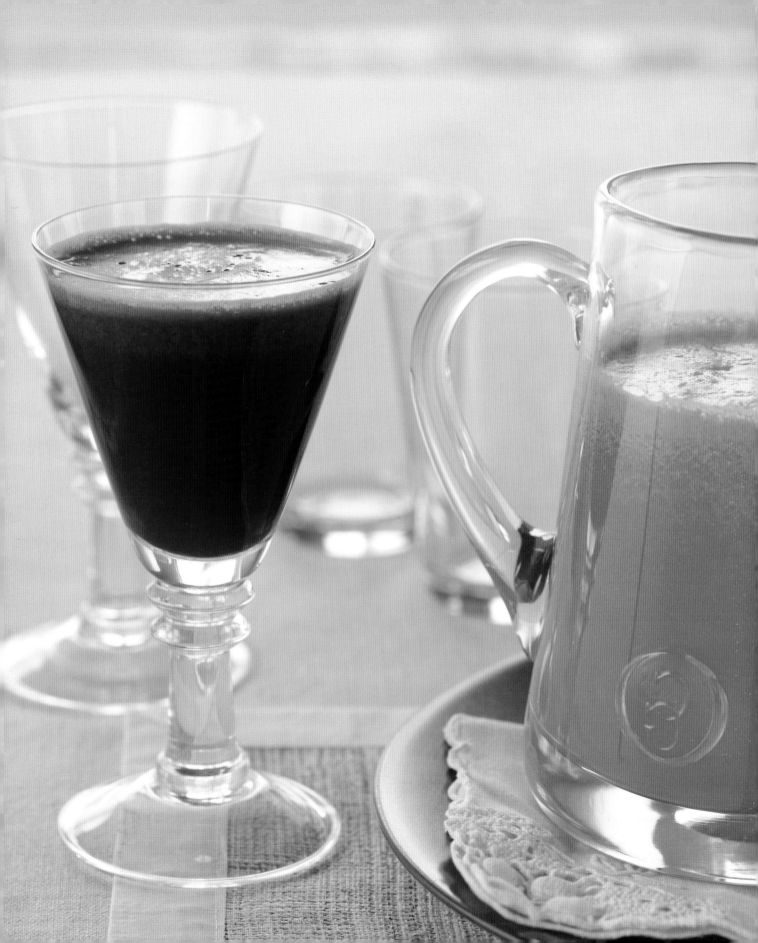

watermelon juice with maca powder
serves 4

¼ seedless watermelon, rind removed and flesh chopped
¼ teaspoon maca powder (see note page 34)

Using an electric juice extractor, juice the watermelon into a jug. Stir in the maca powder until well combined. Pour into serving glasses and serve immediately.

beetroot, celery and ginger juice
serves 1

1 large beetroot, including stalks and leaves, scrubbed
1 large granny smith apple, cored and quartered
1 celery stalk, including leaves
1 fresh ginger slice, or to taste

Using an electric juice extractor, juice the beetroot, apple, celery and ginger into a jug. Pour into a serving glass and serve immediately.

Maca powder is a whole protein from the Amazon rainforest and is a superfood providing strength, endurance and aiding in hormonal balance. It can be added to any juice combination.

shakes, smoothies and juices

carrot, asparagus, parsley and pineapple juice
serves 2

½ pineapple, peeled, cored and
    chopped
60 g (2¼ oz/2 cups) flat-leaf
    (Italian) parsley (use leaves
    and stalks)
175 g (6 oz) asparagus spears
1 large carrot, halved lengthways

Using an electric juice extractor, juice the pineapple, parsley, asparagus and carrot into a jug. Pour into serving glasses and serve immediately.

carrot, broccoli and apple juice
serves 2

2 large carrots, chopped
30 g (1 oz/½ cup) broccoli florets
2 granny smith apples, cored and
    quartered
leaves from 1 small bunch turnips

Using an electric juice extractor, juice the carrot, broccoli, apple and turnip leaves into a jug. Pour into serving glasses and serve immediately.

kale, apple and beetroot juice
serves 2

50 g (1¾ oz/1 cup) kale
2 granny smith apples, cored and
   quartered
1 beetroot, including stalks and
   leaves, scrubbed
¼ red or green cabbage,
   chopped
1 garlic clove

Using an electric juice extractor, juice the kale, apple, beetroot, cabbage and garlic into a jug. Pour into serving glasses and serve immediately.

I love that I can get my greens for the day, plus the beets and of course, an apple a day all in one hit!

spicy carrot, celery and tomato juice
serves 2

2 large carrots, halved lengthways
3 celery stalks, including leaves,
  chopped
1 large tomato, quartered
pinch cayenne pepper

Using an electric juice extractor, juice the carrot, celery and tomato into a jug. Stir in the cayenne pepper until well combined. Pour into serving glasses and serve immediately.

spinach, broccoli and capsicum juice
serves 2

4 large English spinach leaves
30 g (1 oz/½ cup) broccoli florets
1 red capsicum (pepper), seeded,
  membrane removed and
  chopped
2 granny smith apples, cored and
  quartered
1 garlic clove

Using an electric juice extractor, juice the spinach, broccoli, capsicum, apple and garlic into a jug. Pour into serving glasses and serve immediately.

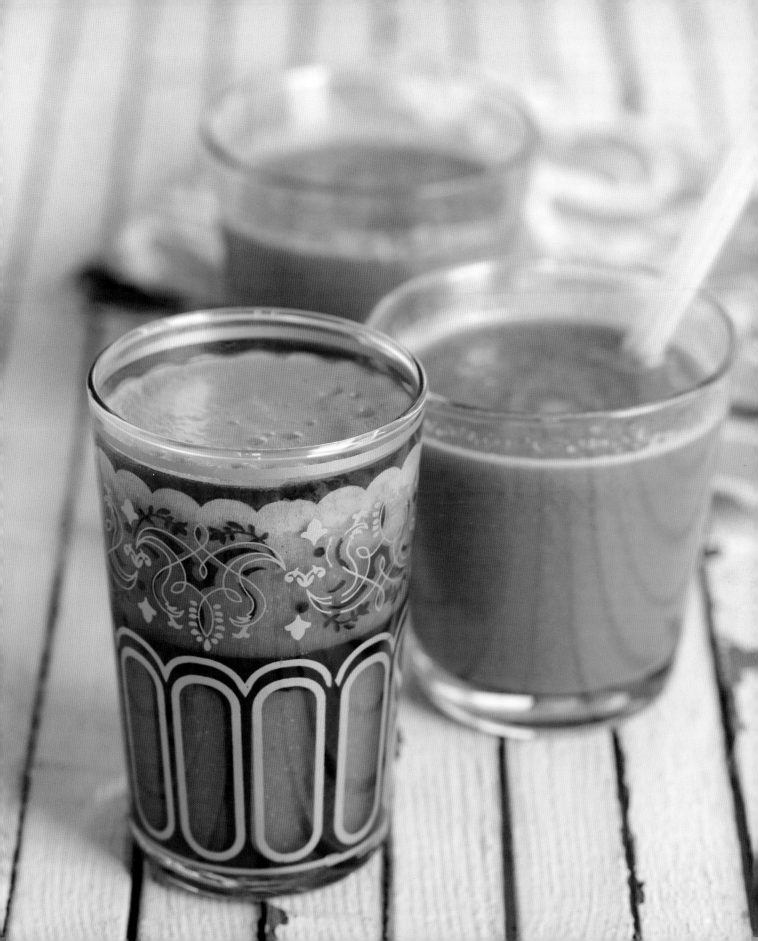

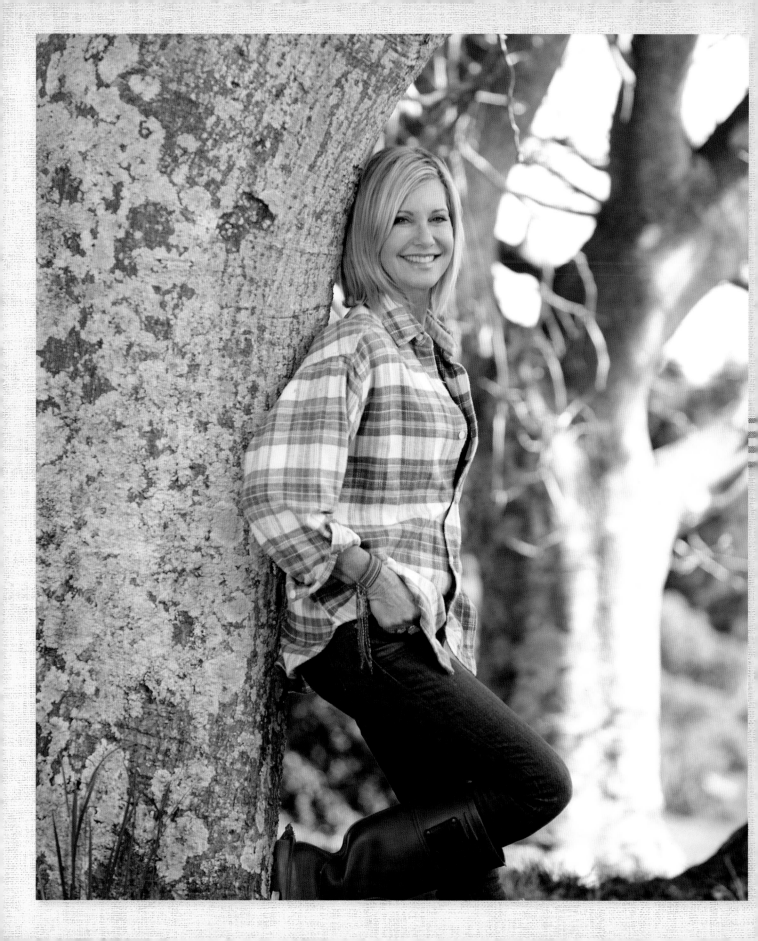

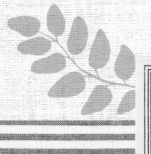

starters, snacks and breads

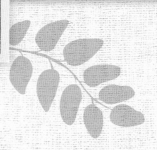

cornbread
makes 1 loaf

400 g (14 oz/2 cups) fresh corn
   kernels
1 teaspoon sea salt
2 tablespoons extra virgin olive oil
150 g (5½ oz/1 cup) polenta
caraway seeds (optional)

Preheat the oven to 180°C (350°F/Gas 4). Line the base and sides of a 12 x 20 x 6 cm (4½ x 8 x 2½ inch) loaf (bar) tin with baking paper.

Put the corn in a food processor with 500 ml (17 fl oz/2 cups) water and process until almost smooth. Transfer to a large bowl and add the salt, olive oil and polenta. Mix together until well combined.

Pour the mixture into the prepared tin and sprinkle the caraway seeds over the top, if using. Bake for 50 minutes, or until a skewer inserted into the centre of the loaf comes out clean. Allow to cool in the tin for 10 minutes, before transferring to a wire rack. Cut into slices and serve the cornbread warm or cold. Serve with your favourite spread or at breakfast with poached eggs, tomatoes, mushrooms and avocado.

This cornbread can be stored, wrapped in plastic wrap, at room temperature for up to 2 days. It can be frozen for up to 3 months. Warm the cornbread slices in a toaster or a preheated oven before serving.

Cornbread makes such a delicious change from wheat breads and can be served with either savoury or sweet toppings.

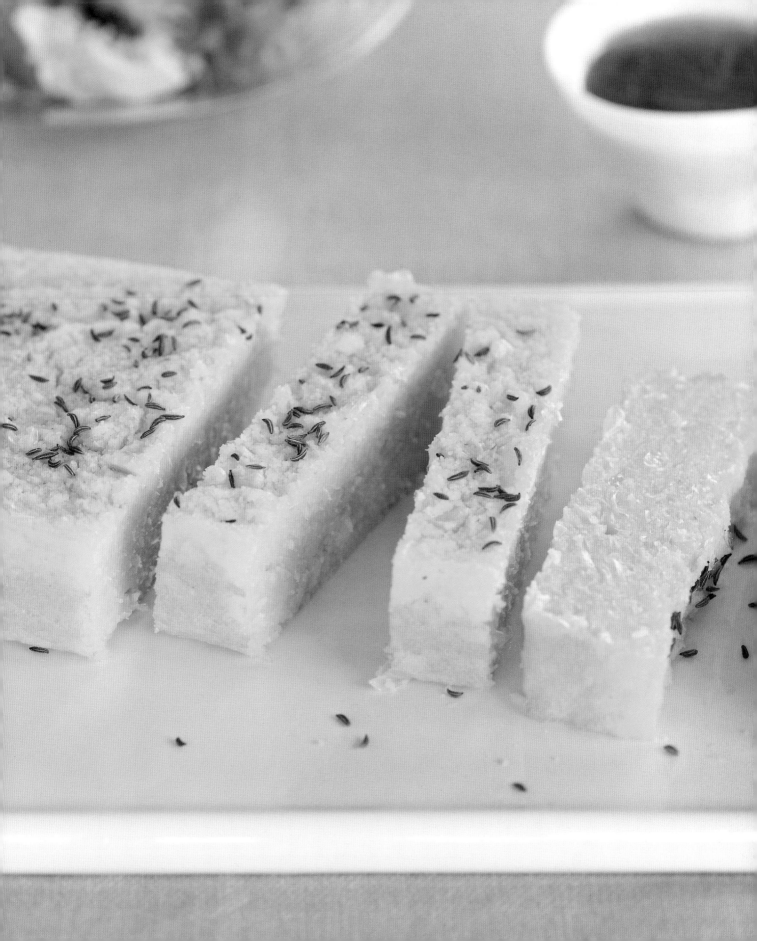

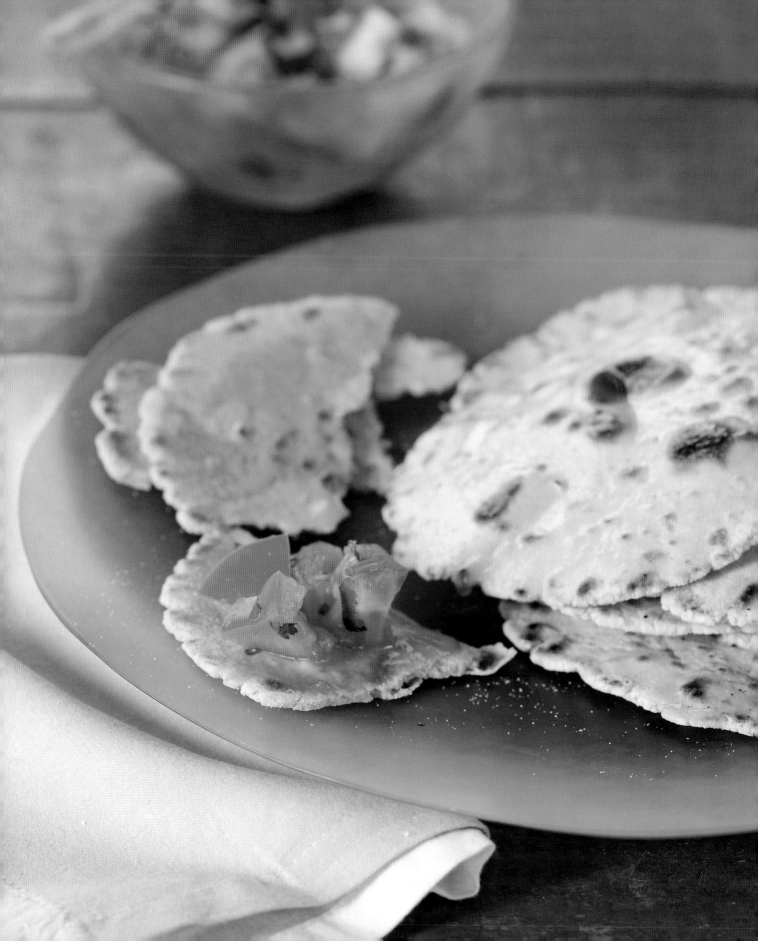

chapatti
makes 12

220 g (7¾ oz/2 cups) besan
   (chickpea) flour
½ teaspoon sea salt
2 tablespoons ghee, melted

Combine the besan flour and salt in a large bowl and make a well in the centre. Stir in 185 ml (6 fl oz/¾ cup) water, or enough to mix to a soft dough. Use your hands to bring the dough together into a ball.

Turn the dough out onto a lightly floured surface and knead until the dough is smooth. Place in a lightly oiled bowl, cover with plastic wrap and set aside for 1 hour.

Divide the dough into 12 even-sized pieces. Use a rolling pin to roll each piece out on a lightly floured work surface to form circles with a 15 cm (6 inch) diameter, about 1 cm (½ inch) thick. Shake off any excess flour and set aside.

Heat a large frying pan over high heat. Brush both sides of the chapatti with the melted ghee and cook, one at a time, for about 1 minute, or until bubbles form on the surface, then turn over and cook for a further 1 minute, or until cooked through. Transfer to a serving plate and keep warm. Repeat with the remaining 11 chapatti.

Serve chapatti warm or at room temperature.

chilled watermelon gazpacho
serves 8–10

1 red capsicum (pepper), seeded, membrane removed and quartered

1 yellow capsicum (pepper), seeded, membrane removed and quartered

3 kg (6 lb 12 oz) seedless watermelon

1 Lebanese (short) cucumber, cut into 5 mm (¼ inch) pieces

3 celery stalks, cut into 5 mm (¼ inch) pieces

½ small red onion, finely chopped

¼ cup mint leaves, finely chopped

150 ml (5 fl oz) freshly squeezed lime juice

60 ml (2 fl oz/¼ cup) red wine vinegar

Preheat the grill (broiler) to high. Place the capsicums, skin side up, on a baking tray and cook under the grill for about 10 minutes, or until the skin blisters and blackens. Place the capsicum in a plastic bag and stand for 10 minutes or until cooled, then peel the skin and finely chop the flesh into 5 mm (¼ inch) pieces.

Finely chop some of the watermelon into 5 mm (¼ inch) cubes and set aside — you need about 1 cup. Combine with the capsicum, cucumber, celery and onion. Cover and refrigerate until required.

Chop the remaining watermelon, put into a blender and blend until smooth — you may need to do this in batches. Transfer to a large bowl and stir in the mint, lime juice and vinegar. Add half of the reserved watermelon and vegetable mixture and stir well to combine. Refrigerate the gazpacho and remaining watermelon and vegetable mixture for at least 1 hour, or until well chilled. Serve in bowls or glasses topped with the remaining watermelon and vegetable mixture.

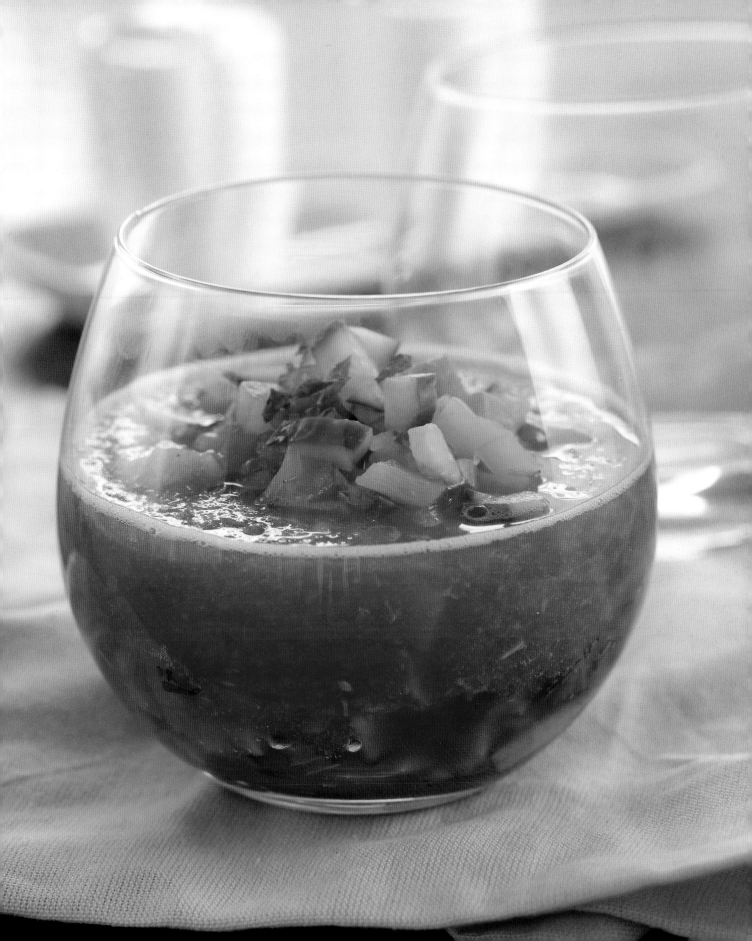

pizza base
makes 1 base

1 cup sprouted wholegrain
   buckwheat, rinsed (see
   pages 14–15)
60 ml (2 fl oz/¼ cup) olive oil
100 g (3½ oz/⅔ cup) soaked and
   drained linseeds
60 ml (2 fl oz/¼ cup) fresh carrot
   juice
140 g (5 oz/1 cup) carrot pulp
1 teaspoon sea salt
1 garlic clove, chopped

Put all of the ingredients in a food processor and process until smooth, adding a little water if necessary — the mixture should resemble a smooth paste.

Spread the mixture evenly over a plastic dehydrator sheet, about 5 mm (¼ inch) thick. Set the dehydrator temperature to high and dehydrate for 1 hour.

Decrease the temperature to medium and continue to dehydrate the base for about 5 hours, or until the top of the base hardens and starts to crack a little. Turn the base over and place back on the dehydrator sheet. Dehydrate for about 5 hours longer, or until the crust is very dry and firm.

This pizza base recipe is good for people with a gluten intolerance — both kids and adults will love it.

davidson plum and goji berry chutney
makes 4 cups

1 kg (2 lb 4 oz) davidson plums or
    regular plums
1 red onion, finely chopped
1 cup rapadura (unprocessed
    sugar) (see notes)
100 g (3½ oz) mixed goji berries
    (see notes) and currants
60 ml (2 fl oz/¼ cup) Japanese
    plum vinegar or cider vinegar
1 garlic clove, crushed
1 bay leaf
1 tablespoon black mustard seeds

Cut the plums in half, remove the stones and coarsely chop the flesh.

Place the plums and all of the other ingredients into a large saucepan over medium heat. Bring to the boil, then reduce the heat to low and simmer, stirring occasionally, for about 30 minutes, or until the mixture has reduced by one-third.

Spoon the chutney into hot sterilised jars, seal and cool. Label and date the jars. The chutney can be stored in a cool dark place for up to 6 months. Refrigerate after opening.

Notes: Rapadura sugar is an unrefined and unbleached whole cane sugar. It is available from health food stores.

Goji berries, also known as wolfberries (*Lycium barbarum*), are the small red berries that are dried and sold in packets. They are available from health food stores.

pesto sauce
makes 4 cups

310 g (11 oz/2 cups) pine nuts,
    toasted
3 bunches fresh basil, leaves picked
2 garlic cloves, quartered
60 ml (2 fl oz/¼ cup) olive oil
freshly squeezed juice of ½ lemon
1 teaspoon sea salt
115 g (4 oz/1 cup) ground hemp
    seeds (see note) or walnuts
1 teaspoon green barley grass
    powder (see note page 50)

Put all of the ingredients into a food processor and process until well combined and smooth.

This pesto can be stored in an airtight container in the refrigerator for up to 3 days.

Note: Hemp seeds are packed with all the essential amino acids and essential fatty acids necessary for a healthy life. They are small nut-brown seeds and are available from health food stores.

starters, snacks and breads

guacamole dip
makes about 2 cups

2 large avocados
½ small red onion, finely chopped
1 large roma (plum) tomato, finely
   chopped
1 garlic clove, crushed
1–2 teaspoons ground cumin, or
   to taste
1–2 teaspoons ground coriander,
   or to taste
freshly squeezed juice of 1 lemon

Halve the avocados, remove the stones and then peel.
Roughly mash the flesh in a large bowl. Add the onion,
tomato, garlic, cumin, coriander and lemon juice and stir well
to combine.

Serve the guacamole with baked potatoes or julienne
vegetables. Guacamole needs to be eaten straight away and
will not store for any length of time.

red kidney bean dip
makes about 3 cups

400 g (14 oz) tin red kidney beans
2 tomatoes, diced
worcestershire sauce, to taste
1 tablespoon tomato paste
   (concentrated purée)
1 red onion, finely chopped
1 garlic clove, crushed
½ teaspoon mild paprika
1 teaspoon sea salt

Put all of the ingredients into a food processor and process
to make a smooth paste. Serve the red kidney bean dip with
organic corn chips.

Red kidney bean dip can be stored in an airtight container in
the refrigerator for 1 day.

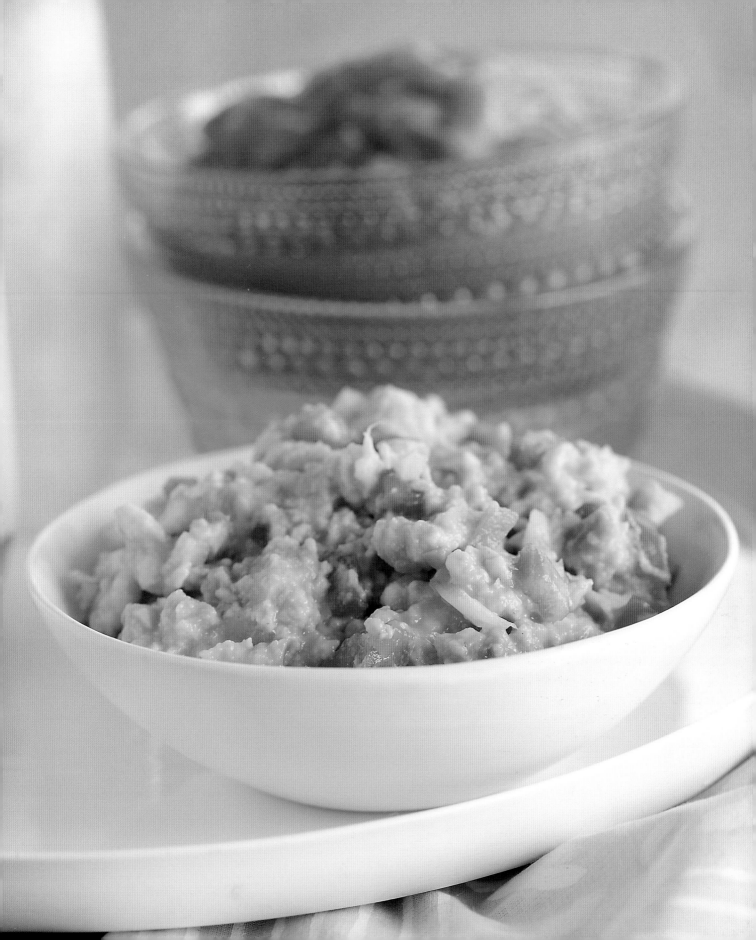

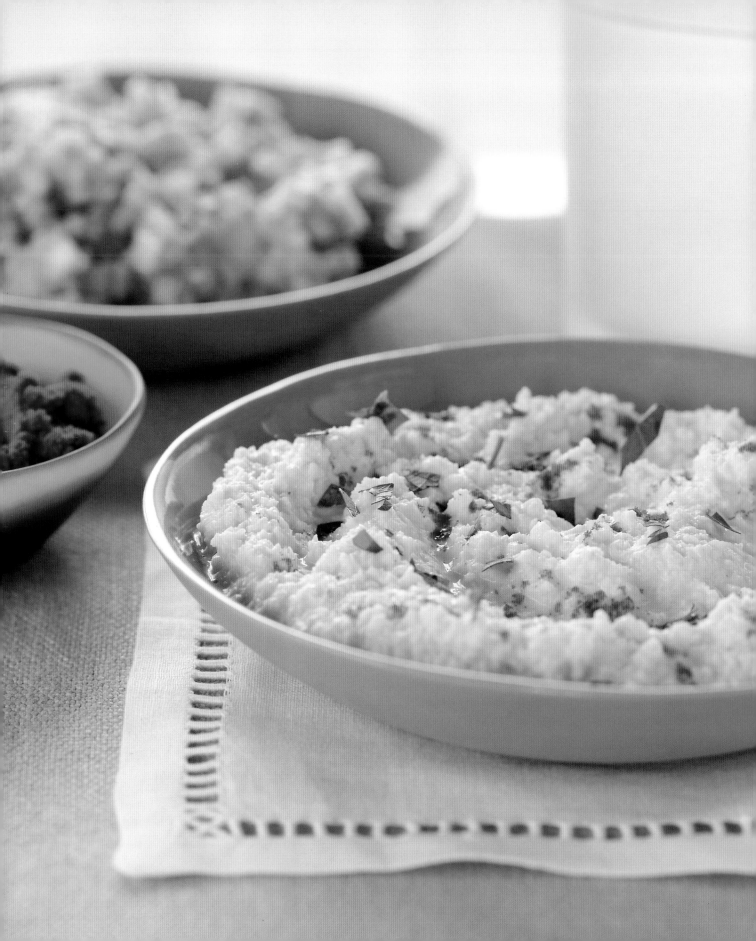

sprouted hummus dip
makes 3 cups

255 g (9 oz/1½ cups) sprouted
   chickpeas (see pages 14–15)
65 g (2¼ oz/¼ cup) tahini
80 ml (2½ fl oz/⅓ cup) olive oil
250 ml (9 fl oz/1 cup) freshly
   squeezed lemon juice
3 garlic cloves, crushed
1 teaspoon sea salt
1 teaspoon mild paprika, to serve
2 tablespoons finely chopped
   flat-leaf (Italian) parsley,
   to serve

Put the sprouted chickpeas into a heatproof bowl and pour
over 750 ml (26 fl oz/3 cups) boiling water. Set aside for at
least 1 minute (this is an important step and will greatly
enhance the flavour of the hummus). Drain well.

Put the sprouted chickpeas, tahini, 60 ml (2 fl oz/¼ cup) of the
olive oil, lemon juice, garlic and salt in a food processor and
process until smooth.

Serve the sprouted hummus dip in a bowl with the remaining
oil drizzled over the top. Sprinkle over the paprika and
parsley, to garnish.

Note: To make a beetroot hummus, omit the chickpeas and
add 3–4 cooked baby beetroot to the food processor with
the remaining ingredients and process until smooth.

avocado salsa
makes 2 cups

1 large avocado
2 garlic cloves, crushed
1 small red onion, finely chopped
freshly squeezed juice of ½ lemon
1 teaspoon sea salt

Halve the avocado, remove the stone and then peel. Coarsely
mash the flesh in a bowl. Add the garlic, onion, lemon juice
and salt and stir well to combine.

Serve the avocado salsa with organic corn chips. The salsa is
best eaten on the day it is made.

vegan cream cheese
makes 1½–2 cups

155 g (5½ oz/1 cup) cashews
80 g (2¾ oz/½ cup) blanched
almonds
¼ teaspoon sea salt
freshly squeezed juice of 1 lemon

Wash the cashews and almonds under cold running water and drain well. Place in a bowl, cover with cold water and leave to soak overnight. Drain well.

Put all of the ingredients into a food processor with 185 ml (6 fl oz/¾ cup) water and process until the mixture is well combined and smooth.

Transfer the mixture to a squeeze bottle as this will help when serving. Drizzle it over pizza Italiano (see page 123) or use it to dress a salad.

Vegan cream cheese can be stored in an airtight container in the refrigerator for up to 10 days.

vegan parmesan cheese
makes about 1 cup

155 g (5½ oz) Brazil nuts or
hazelnuts
1 garlic clove, chopped
1 pinch sea salt

Put all of the ingredients into a food processor and process until finely chopped.

Vegan parmesan cheese is used in the salad topping on the pizza Italiano (see page 123), or can be added to any basic salad. It can be stored in an airtight container in the freezer for up to 3 months.

cracker bread
makes about 20 pieces

125 g (4½ oz/1½ cups) sprouted
   wheat (see page 14–15)
1 teaspoon sea salt

Put the sprouted wheat, sea salt and 60 ml (2 fl oz/¼ cup) water in a food processor and process to make a smooth paste, adding more water if necessary.

Pour the mixture evenly over plastic dehydrator sheets. Set the dehydrator temperature to low. Place in the dehydrator and dehydrate for about 24 hours, or until the bread lifts away from the dehydrator sheets.

Note: You can sprinkle your favourite herbs, seeds or spices over the top of cracker breads before baking. Cracker bread can be stored in an airtight container for up to 1 week.

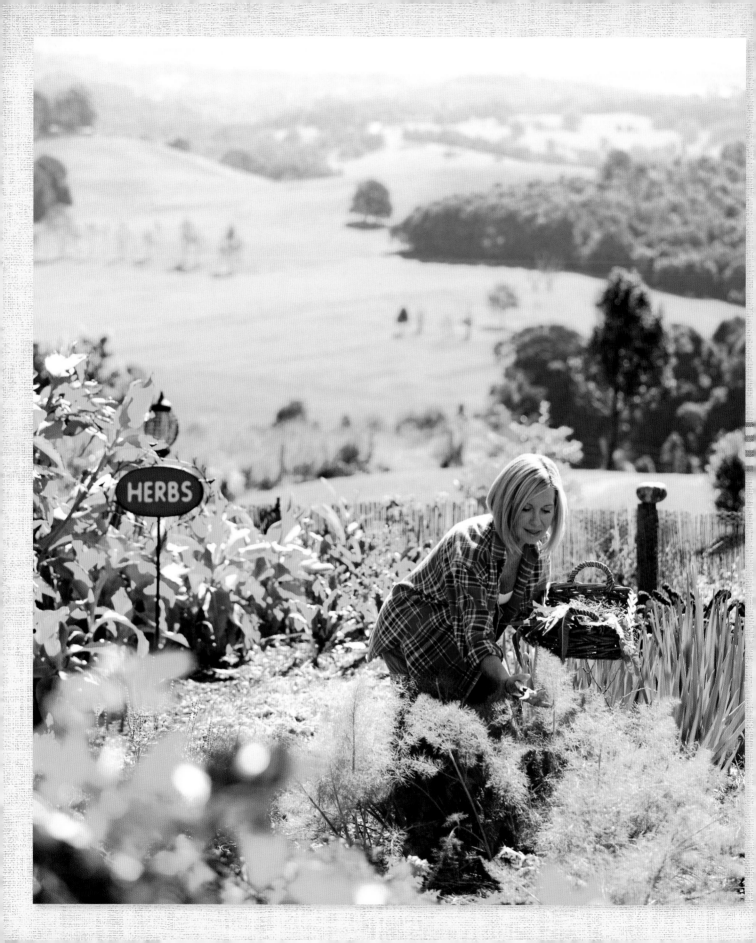

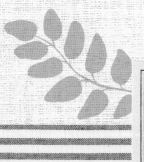

salads and dressings

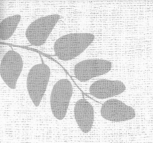

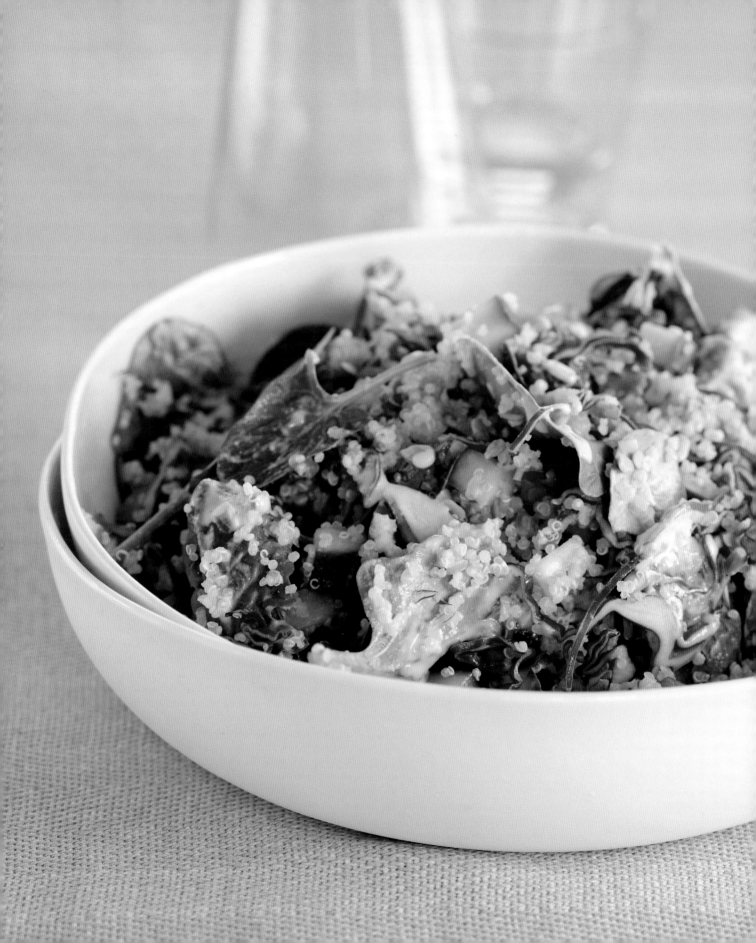

quinoa salad
serves 4

200 g (7 oz/1 cup) quinoa

60 g (2¼ oz//½ cup) sunflower
seeds

1 tablespoon tamari or soy sauce

2 Lebanese (short) cucumbers,
diced

80 g (2¾ oz/1 cup) shredded red
cabbage

4 spring onions (scallions), thinly
sliced

80 g (2¾ oz/1¾ cups) baby
spinach leaves

SPICY TAHINI DRESSING

65 g (2½ oz/¼ cup) tahini

freshly squeezed juice of 1 lemon

1 tablespoon white miso paste

2 garlic cloves, crushed

pinch cayenne pepper

To make the spicy tahini dressing, put all of the ingredients into a small bowl with 60 ml (2 fl oz/¼ cup) water. Whisk well until smooth and combined. Set aside until needed.

Put the quinoa and 500 ml (17 fl oz/2 cups) water in a small saucepan over high heat. Bring to the boil, then reduce the heat to low, cover, and simmer for 10–15 minutes, or until the quinoa is tender and all of the water has been absorbed. Remove from the heat, transfer to a large bowl and cool.

Meanwhile, dry-fry the sunflower seeds in a frying pan over medium heat for 1 minute, or until aromatic. Add the tamari to the pan, then remove from the heat and stir well to coat the seeds. Add to the quinoa with the cucumber, cabbage, spring onion and spinach and toss gently to combine. Drizzle over the spicy tahini dressing and toss well before serving.

Salads are a staple at my house — I always keep salad supplies in the fridge so I can whip up an easy lunch at short notice.

coleslaw with cashew nut dressing
serves 4

¼ red cabbage, shredded
¼ green cabbage, shredded
2 large carrots, grated
2 celery stalks, thinly sliced
1 red capsicum (pepper), seeded,
    membrane removed and sliced
1 large red onion, thinly sliced
100 g (3½ oz) chopped pineapple

CASHEW NUT DRESSING
80 g (2¾ oz/½ cup) cashew nuts
freshly squeezed juice of ½ lemon
½ teaspoon garlic powder (see note)
pinch sea salt

To make the cashew nut dressing, soak the cashews in 125 ml (4 fl oz/½ cup) water for at least 1 hour. Drain well.

Put the cashews into a food processor with the remaining ingredients and process until well combined and almost smooth. Set aside until needed.

Just before you are ready to serve, put all of the salad ingredients and the dressing into a large serving bowl and toss gently to combine.

Note: Garlic powder is made from ground dehyrdated garlic. It is available from most health food stores.

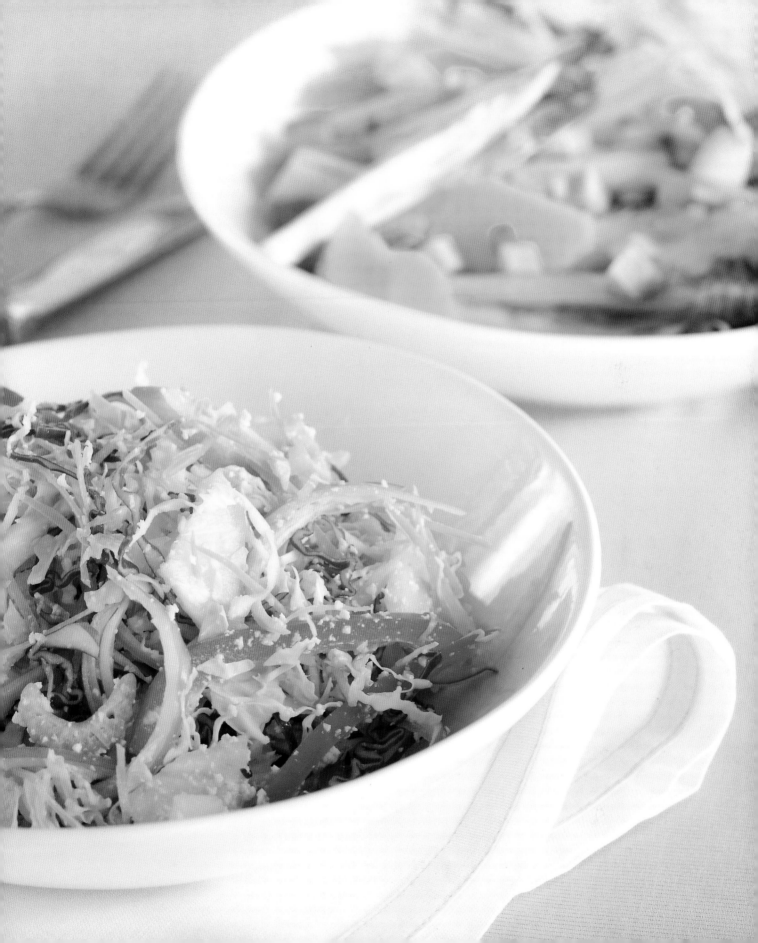

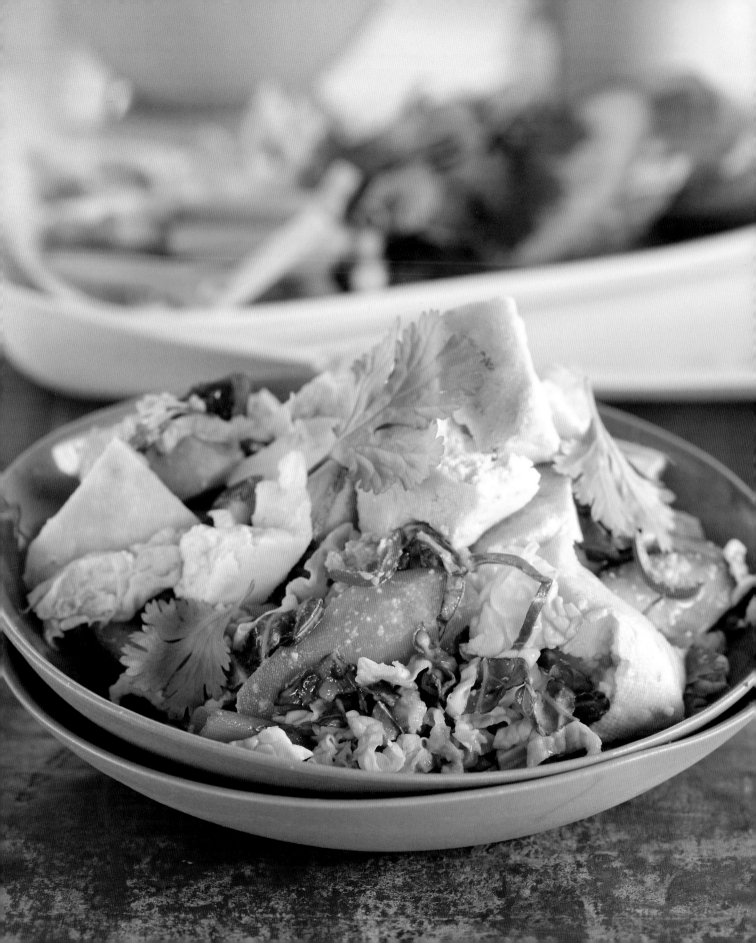

gaia gado gado salad
serves 6

600 g (1 lb 5 oz) firm tofu, cut into
   1 cm (½ inch) cubes
2 lemongrass stems, white part
   only, thinly sliced
2 garlic cloves, lightly crushed
60 ml (2 fl oz/¼ cup) macadamia oil
1 large carrot, thinly sliced
¼ Chinese cabbage (wong bok),
   shredded
500 g (1 lb 2 oz) baby bok choy
   (pak choy), shredded
1 Lebanese (short) cucumber, sliced
½ pineapple, peeled, cored and
   chopped
3 spring onions (scallions), sliced
1 cup coriander (cilantro) leaves
4 long red chillies, seeded and
   thinly sliced

GADO GADO DRESSING
120 g (4¼ oz/¾ cup) macadamia
   nuts or peanuts, lightly toasted
freshly squeezed juice of 3 limes
80 ml (2½ fl oz/⅓ cup) kecap manis
80 ml (2½ fl oz/⅓ cup) coconut milk
1 tablespoon fish sauce
1 garlic clove, crushed

Put the tofu, lemongrass, garlic and macadamia oil into a bowl. Cover with plastic wrap and refrigerate overnight.

To make the gado gado dressing, put the macadamia nuts into a food processor and process until they resemble fine breadcrumbs. Transfer to a bowl and stir in the lime juice, kecap manis, coconut milk, fish sauce and garlic. Set aside until needed.

Cook the carrot in a small saucepan of boiling water for 2 minutes, or until tender. Refresh in cold water, drain well and set aside.

Cook the tofu on a hot barbecue plate or in a frying pan over medium heat for 2–3 minutes, turning often, until golden brown — the lemongrass should be a little crunchy.

Put the carrot and remaining salad ingredients into a large bowl and toss well to combine. Add the gado gado dressing and gently toss again before serving. Place the tofu on top.

garden salad
serves 2

½ red capsicum (pepper), halved
    seeded and membrane removed
2 teaspoons olive oil
2 garlic cloves, crushed
80 g (2¾ oz/2 cups) mixed salad
    leaves
1 carrot, coarsely grated
1 beetroot, trimmed, peeled and
    coarsely grated
6 cherry tomatoes, halved
¼ red onion, thinly sliced
4 semi-dried (sun-blushed)
    tomatoes, chopped
1 avocado, peeled, stone
    removed and flesh diced
½ cup mung bean sprouts
¼ cup basil, mint or Italian (flat-
    leaf) parsley, finely chopped
salad dressing of your choice,
    to serve (see pages 102–107)

Preheat the oven to 200°C (400°F/Gas 6). Line a baking tray with baking paper.

Place the capsicum quarters on the prepared tray. Drizzle with the oil and sprinkle with garlic. Bake for 20 minutes, or until tender. When cool enough to handle, cut the capsicum into thick strips.

Divide the capsicum and remaining ingredients between two serving bowls and toss gently to combine. Drizzle the dressing over the salad and serve immediately.

Note: Try adding some crumbled goat's cheese or fresh mozzarella cheese for extra flavour — delicious!

My husband, John, calls my salads 'kitchen roulette' because I never make them the same way twice! I tend to use whatever is in the fridge and just add one of my favourite dressings.

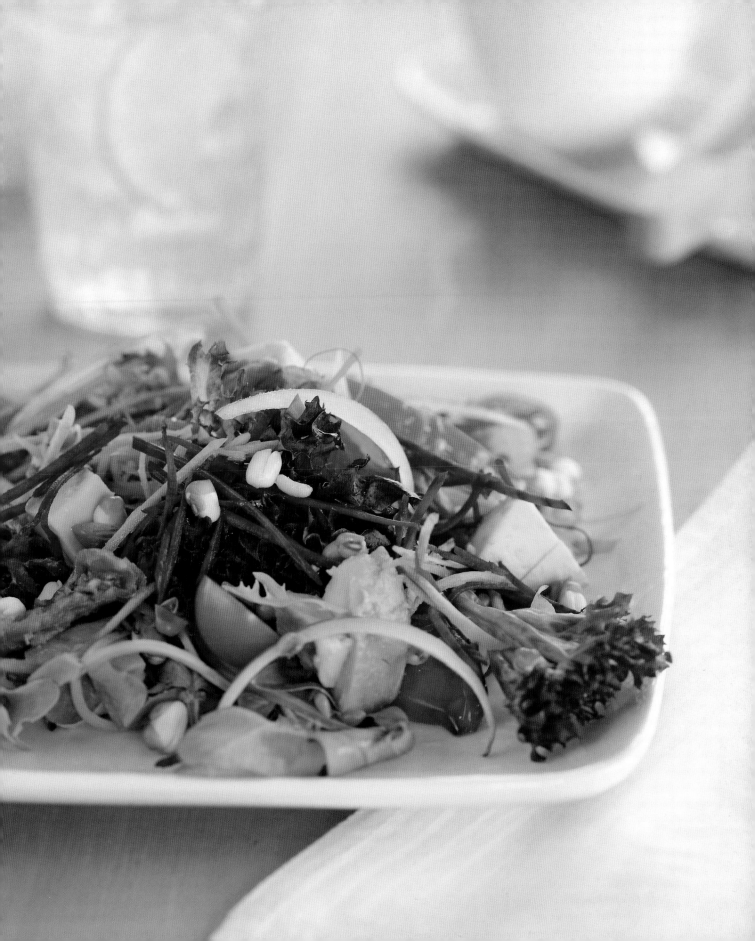

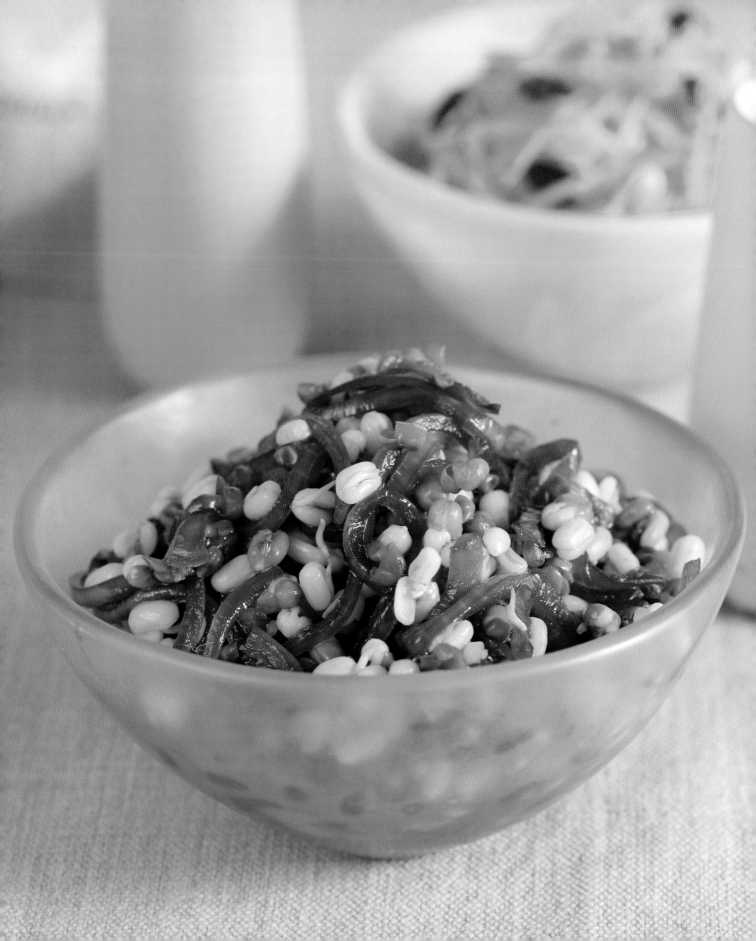

mung bean salad
serves 2

185 g (6½ oz/2 cups) mung bean
   sprouts
2 teaspoons coconut oil (see note
   page 36)
1 large brown onion, thinly sliced
2 garlic cloves, crushed
1 teaspoon grated fresh ginger
60 ml (2 fl oz/¼ cup) shoyu
   (Japanese soy sauce)
1½ tablespoons brown rice vinegar
   (see note)
1 teaspoon sesame oil

Put the mung bean sprouts in a colander and pour boiling
water over them. Drain well.

Heat the coconut oil in a large frying pan over medium–high
heat. Cook the onion, garlic and ginger for about 5 minutes,
or until softened. Add the shoyu, rice vinegar and sesame
oil and cook for a further 2 minutes, stirring well to combine.
Remove from the heat and stir in the sprouts. Transfer to a
serving bowl and serve immediately.

Note: You can also serve this salad on a bed of steamed rice
or with lightly pan-fried tofu.

Brown rice vinegar is available from health food stores.

carrot salad with papaya and orange dressing
serves 2

2 large carrots, coarsely grated
50 g (1¾ oz/⅓ cup) pine nuts,
   toasted
40 g (1½ oz/⅓ cup) sultanas
   (golden raisins)

PAPAYA AND ORANGE DRESSING
185 g (6½ oz/1 cup) chopped red
   papaya
125 ml (4 fl oz/½ cup) freshly
   squeezed orange juice
125 ml (4 fl oz/½ cup) olive oil
pinch sea salt

To make the papaya and orange dressing place all of the
ingredients into a blender and blend until smooth. Set aside
until needed.

Put all of the salad ingredients and the dressing into a large
serving bowl and toss gently to combine. Serve immediately.

tomato and bocconcini salad
with raspberry vinaigrette
serves 4

8 heirloom tomatoes, cut into
   wedges
30 g (1 oz/1 cup) watercress
50 g (1¾ oz) rocket (arugula)
   leaves
2 spring onions (scallions), thinly
   sliced
¼ cup chopped mixed herbs,
   such as flat-leaf (Italian) parsley
   and basil
4 bocconcini, quartered

RASPBERRY VINAIGRETTE
80 ml (2½ fl oz/⅓ cup) extra
   virgin olive oil
30 ml (1 fl oz) raspberry vinegar
½ teaspoon dijon mustard
1 small garlic clove, crushed

To make the raspberry vinaigrette, combine all of the ingredients in a jar and shake well to combine.

Put the tomato in a bowl and drizzle over the vinaigrette. Set aside for at least 5 minutes.

Add the remaining salad ingredients to the bowl and gently toss before serving.

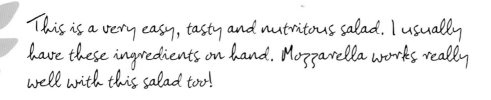

This is a very easy, tasty and nutritous salad. I usually have these ingredients on hand. Mozzarella works really well with this salad too!

papaya and avocado salad with lime ginger dressing

serves 2

185 g (6½ oz/4 cups) chopped witlof (chicory/Belgian endive)
360 g (12¾ oz) red papaya, sliced
1 large avocado, peeled, stone removed and flesh diced
2 spring onions (scallions), sliced

LIME GINGER DRESSING
60 ml (2 fl oz/¼ cup) olive oil
60 ml (2 fl oz/¼ cup) freshly squeezed lime juice
1 tablespoon finely grated fresh ginger
¼ teaspoon mild curry powder

To make the lime ginger dressing, combine all of the ingredients in a jar and shake well to combine. Set aside until needed.

Put all of the salad ingredients into a large bowl and toss gently to combine. Drizzle over the lime ginger dressing and toss to coat before serving.

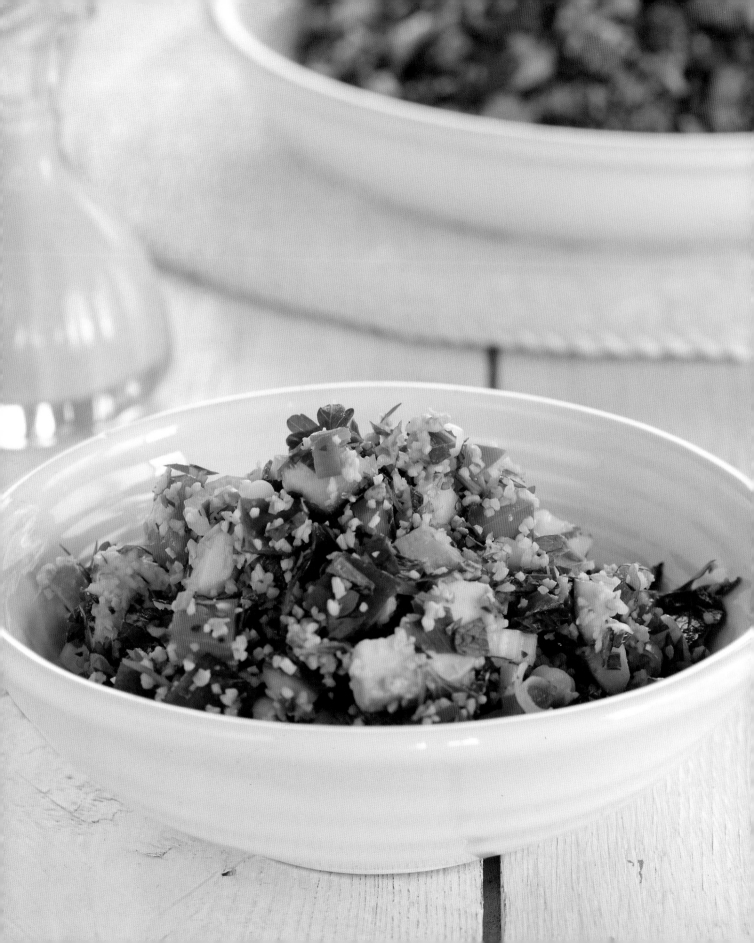

tabouleh and avocado salad

serves 4

90 g (3¼ oz/½ cup) burghul
(bulgur)

1 celery stalk, thinly sliced

1 Lebanese (short) cucumber, cut
into 1 cm (½ inch) cubes

2 large roma (plum) tomatoes,
seeded and cut into 1 cm
(½ inch) cubes

2 large avocados, peeled, stones
removed and flesh thinly sliced

8 spring onions (scallions), thinly
sliced

1 bunch flat-leaf (Italian) parsley,
leaves finely chopped

1 bunch mint, leaves finely
chopped

LEMON VINEGAR DRESSING
125 ml (4 fl oz/½ cup) olive oil
freshly squeezed juice of 2 lemons
finely grated zest of 2 lemons
2 tablespoons white wine vinegar
1 garlic clove, crushed
pinch sea salt
pinch xylitol (see note page 33)
2 teaspoons dijon mustard
(optional)

Put the burghul in a bowl and pour over enough boiling water to cover by 5 cm (2 inches). Set aside to soak for 10–15 minutes, or until tender. Drain well.

Meanwhile, to make the lemon vinegar dressing put all of the ingredients into a jar and shake well to combine. Set aside until needed.

Put the drained burghul in a large bowl with the celery, cucumber, tomato, avocado, spring onion, parsley and mint. Add 80 ml (2½ fl oz/⅓ cup) of the lemon vinegar dressing and toss gently to combine.

Divide the salad between serving bowls and drizzle with the remaining dressing, to serve.

pumpkin and beetroot salad with mustard dressing

serves 4

1.25 kg (2 lb 12 oz) baby
  beetroot (beets)
1 tablespoon olive oil
400 g (14 oz) butternut pumpkin
  (squash)
50 g (1¾ oz/½ cup) walnuts,
  toasted
150 g (5½ oz/4 cups) mixed salad
  leaves
80 g (2¾ oz/1¾ cups) baby
  spinach leaves
1 Lebanese (short) cucumber,
  halved lengthways and sliced
8 cherry tomatoes, halved
1 cup basil
4 spring onions (scallions), thinly
  sliced
90 g (3¼ oz/½ cup) sunflower
  sprouts

MUSTARD DRESSING
80 ml (2½ fl oz/⅓ cup) olive oil
2 tablespoons white vinegar
3 teaspoons honey
1 teaspoon wholegrain mustard
1 teaspoon dijon mustard

Preheat the oven to 160°C (315°F/Gas 2–3).

Trim the beetroot leaves, leaving 2 cm (¾ inch) of the stems attached. Gently scrub the beetroot bulbs and pat dry with paper towels. Put into a large bowl, drizzle with half of the olive oil and toss to coat. Wrap each beetroot in foil, place in a large roasting tin and bake for 1 hour, or until tender when tested with a skewer.

Meanwhile, peel the pumpkin, discarding the seeds and cut into small wedges. Place in a roasting tin and lightly coat in the remaining oil. Bake for 25–30 minutes, or until tender and lightly golden.

To make the mustard dressing, combine all of the ingredients in a jar and shake well to combine.

Put the walnuts, salad leaves, spinach, cucumber, tomato, basil, spring onion and sunflower sprouts into a large bowl. Add the mustard dressing and toss well to coat. Serve the salad with the roasted beetroot and pumpkin.

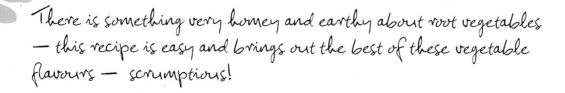

There is something very homey and earthy about root vegetables — this recipe is easy and brings out the best of these vegetable flavours — scrumptious!

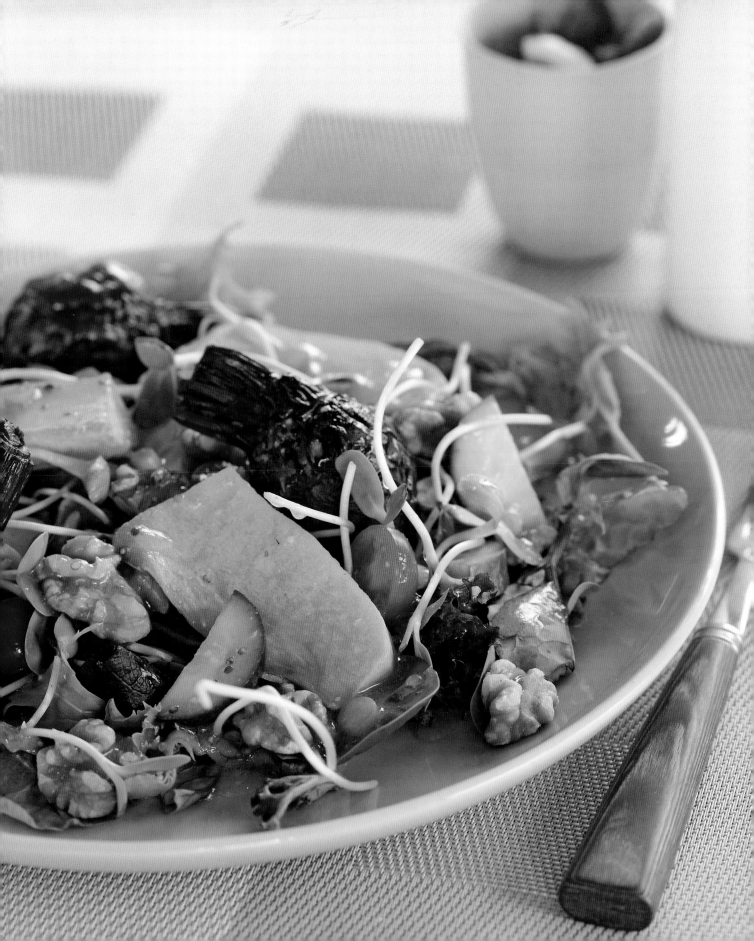

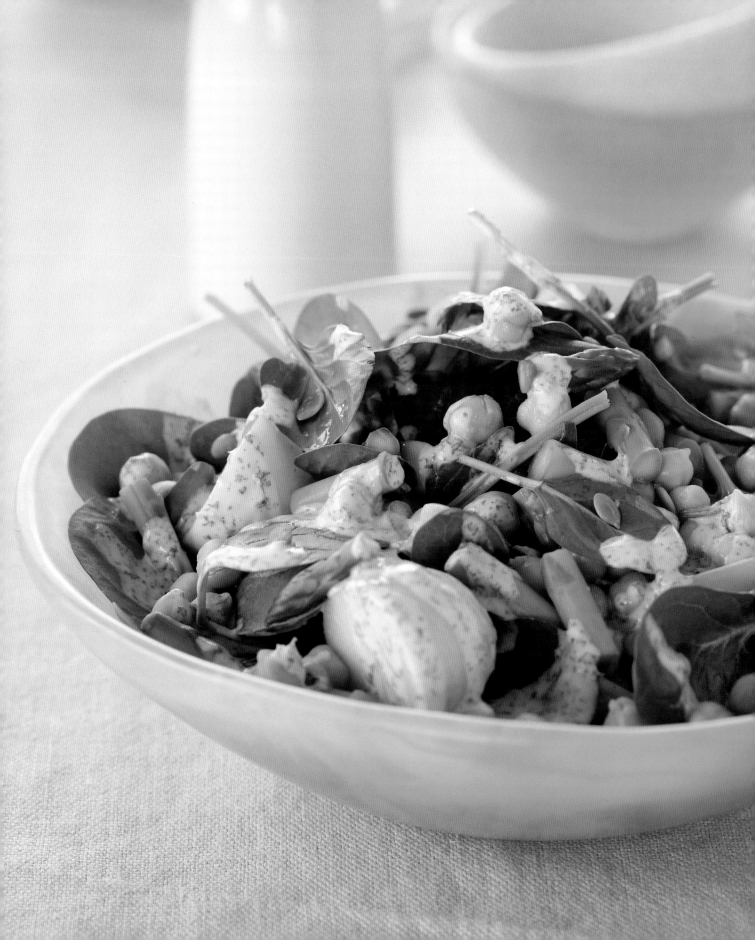

asparagus, chickpea and potato salad with yoghurt and mint dressing

serves 2

150 g (5½ oz) small new potatoes

175 g (6 oz) asparagus spears, trimmed and cut into 3 cm (1¼ inch) lengths

135 g (4¾ oz/3 cups) baby spinach leaves

400 g (14 oz) tin chickpeas, rinsed and drained

30 g (1 oz/¼ cup) pepitas (pumpkin seeds), toasted

YOGHURT AND MINT DRESSING

60 g (2¼ oz/¼ cup) sheep's milk yoghurt

finely grated zest of ½ lime

freshly squeezed juice of ½ lime

freshly squeezed juice of ½ lemon

¼ cup mint leaves, finely chopped

pinch sea salt

To make the yoghurt and mint dressing, put all of the ingredients into a blender and blend until smooth. Cover with plastic wrap and place in the refrigerator until needed.

Cook the potatoes in a large saucepan of boiling water for 10 minutes, or until tender. Add the asparagus to the pan for the last 2 minutes and cook until bright green and tender. Rinse the asparagus immediately under cold water and drain well. Cut the potatoes in half and cool.

Put the spinach, chickpeas, pepitas, asparagus, potato halves and dressing in a large serving bowl and toss gently to combine. Serve immediately with the yoghurt and mint dressing drizzled over the top.

This yoghurt and mint dressing also tastes great spooned over baked potatoes — a whole meal in itself!

green papaya salad
serves 4

1 green papaya, flesh chopped

2 small roma (plum) tomatoes, diced

80 g (2¾ oz/½ cup) macadamia nuts, chopped

¼ teaspoon cayenne pepper

2 tablespoons finely chopped coriander (cilantro) leaves

DRESSING

freshly squeezed juice of ½ lemon

3 garlic cloves, crushed

1 tablespoon shoyu (Japanese soy sauce)

1 tablespoon agave syrup (see note page 22)

To make the dressing, put all of the ingredients into a jar and shake until well combined. Set aside until needed.

Just before you are ready to serve, put all of the salad ingredients into a large serving bowl with the dressing and toss gently to combine. Serve immediately.

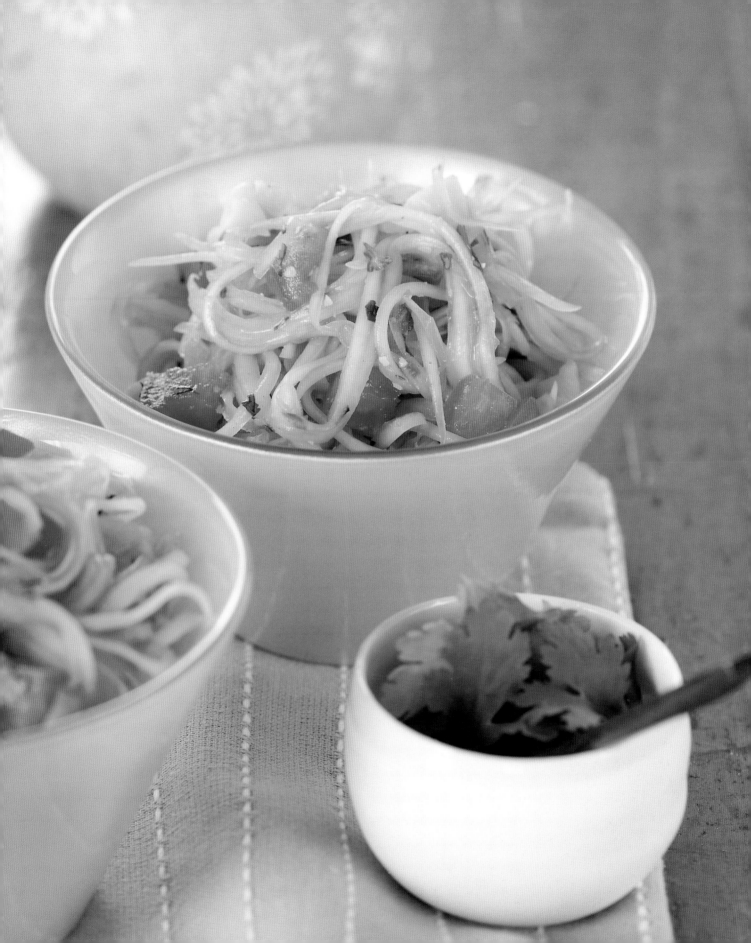

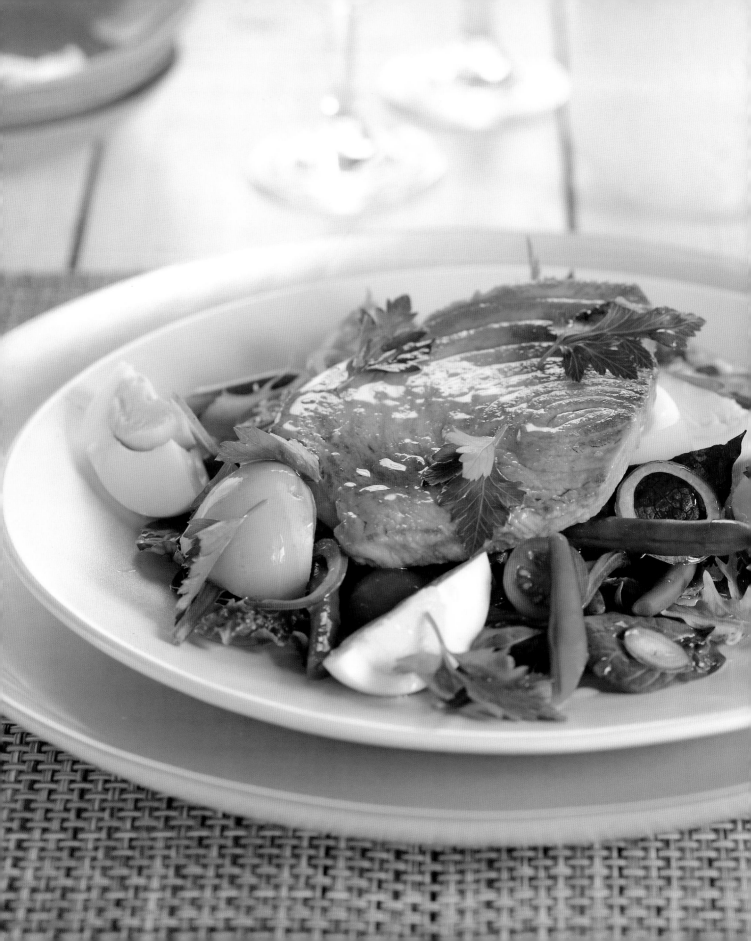

serves 2

150 g (5½ oz) small new potatoes
125 g (4½ oz) green beans
2 x 125 g (4½ oz) tuna steaks
olive oil spray, for cooking
1 small red onion, thinly sliced
2 hard-boiled free-range eggs,
    quartered
80 g (2¾ oz/2 cups) mixed salad
    leaves
8 cherry tomatoes, halved
flat-leaf (Italian) parsley,
    to garnish

OLIVIA'S FAVOURITE DRESSING
freshly squeezed juice of ½ lemon
2 tablespoons olive oil
½ teaspoon Bragg Liquid Aminos,
    or to taste (see note)

To make Olivia's favourite dressing, put the lemon juice, olive oil and the Bragg Liquid Aminos in a jar and shake well to combine. Taste and add more liquid aminos if preferred. Set aside until needed.

Cook the potatoes in a large saucepan of boiling water for 10 minutes, or until bright green and tender. Add the beans to the pan for the last 2 minutes of cooking, or until tender. Rinse the beans immediately under cold water and drain well. Halve the potatoes and set aside to cool.

Spray both sides of the tuna with the oil spray. Sear the tuna on a hot barbecue plate for 2 minutes on each side for medium, or until cooked to your liking. Transfer to a plate and set aside to rest for 2–3 minutes.

Arrange the potato halves on serving plates with the beans, onion, egg, salad leaves and tomato. Top with the tuna and drizzle the dressing over the top. Garnish with the parsley, to serve.

Note: Bragg Liquid Aminos is a Certified non-GMO liquid protein concentrate. It is made from soya beans and contains essential and non-essential amino acids. It is available from most health food stores.

You can replace the tuna steaks in this recipe with a 425 g (15 oz) tin of tuna in springwater or olive oil. Drain well and flake into large chunks before adding to the salad.

basic vinaigrette

makes 170 ml (5½ fl oz/⅔ cup)

60 ml (2 fl oz/¼ cup) olive oil

60 ml (2 fl oz/¼ cup) white wine vinegar

1 tablespoon dijon or wholegrain mustard

1 garlic clove, crushed

1 tablespoon finely chopped flat-leaf (Italian) parsley, oregano or rosemary

Put all of the ingredients into a jar and shake well to combine.

Any leftover dressing can be stored in an airtight container in the refrigerator for up to 1 week.

gaia classic vinaigrette dressing

makes 170 ml (5½ fl oz/⅔ cup)

60 ml (2 fl oz/¼ cup) apple cider vinegar

60 ml (2 fl oz/¼ cup) olive, macadamia, grapeseed or sunflower oil

1 tablespoon dijon or wholegrain mustard

1 tablespoon honey or agave syrup (see note page 22)

Put all of the ingredients into a jar and shake well to combine.

Any leftover dressing can be stored in an airtight container in the refrigerator for up to 10 days.

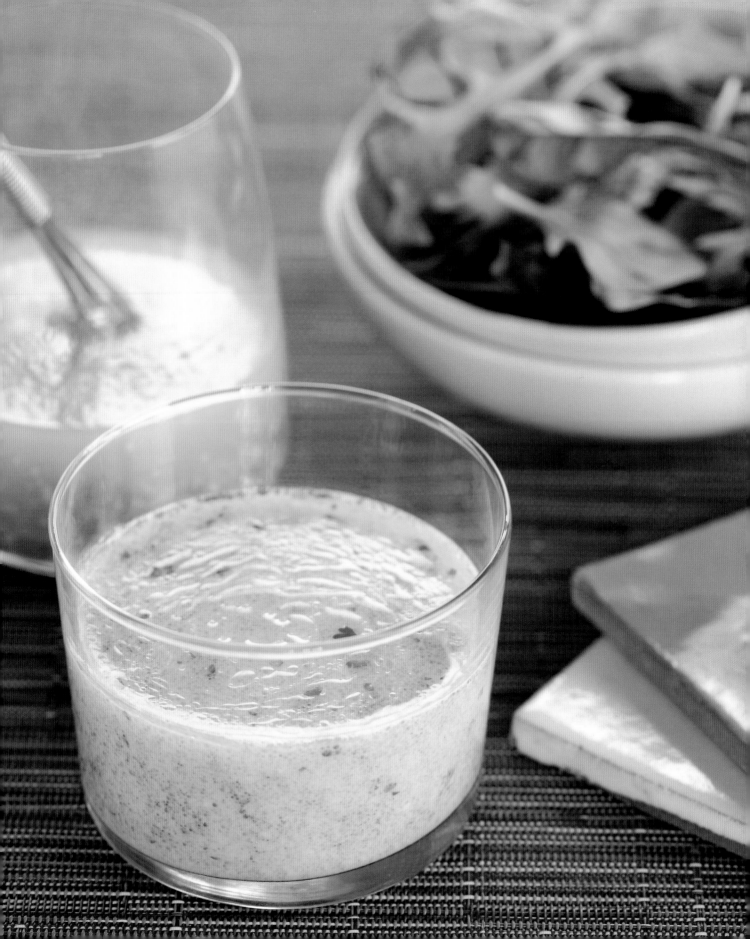

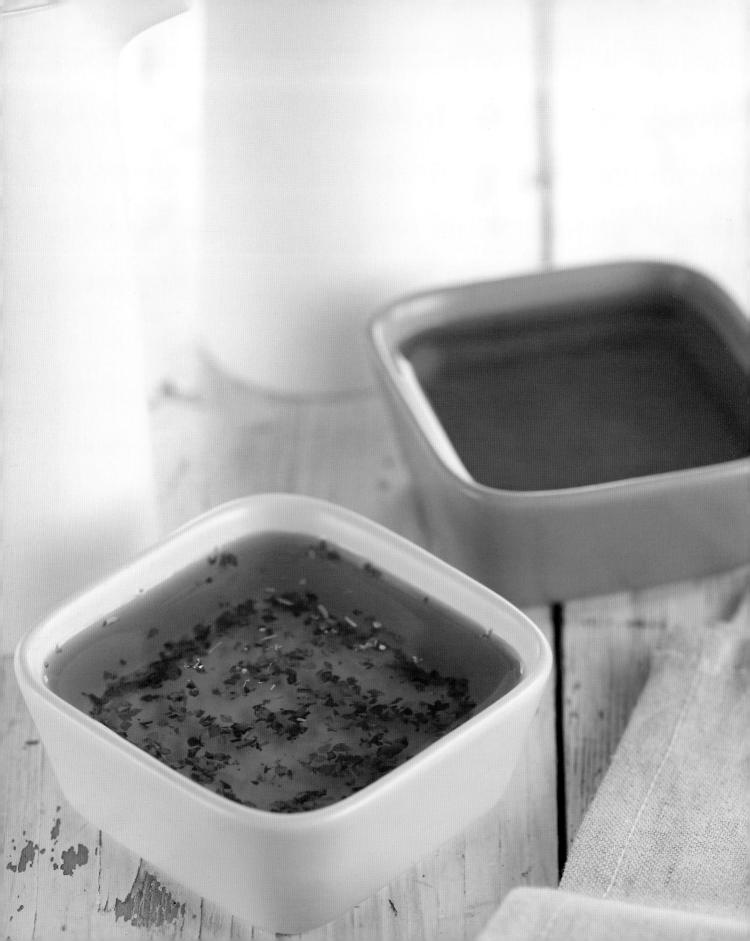

gaia raspberry vinaigrette
makes 125 ml (4 fl oz/½ cup)

1½ tablespoons raspberry vinegar
1½ tablespoons verjuice (see note)
80 ml (2½ fl oz/⅓ cup) macadamia or grapeseed oil

Put all of the ingredients into a jar and shake well to combine.

Any leftover dressing can be stored in an airtight container in the refrigerator for up to 2 weeks.

Note: Verjuice is a milder form of vinegar. It is made from unripened grapes and adds fruity undertones. It is available from most speciality grocery stores and delicatessens.

white wine vinegar and olive oil dressing
makes 250 ml (9 fl oz/1 cup)

80 ml (2½ fl oz/⅓ cup) white wine vinegar
170 ml (5½ fl oz/⅔ cup) olive oil
½ teaspoon dried oregano

Put all of the ingredients into a jar and shake well to combine.

Any leftover dressing can be stored in an airtight container in the refrigerator for up to 1 week.

My husband, John, is a 'sauceaholic' — he gets very excited about the tasty addition that salad dressings and vinaigrettes add to our mealtimes.

soy and sesame dressing
makes 185 ml (6 fl oz/¾ cup)

freshly squeezed juice of 1 lemon
60 ml (2 fl oz/¼ cup) almond oil
1 teaspoon sesame oil
1 garlic clove, crushed
2 tablespoons shoyu (Japanese
  soy sauce)
2 tablespoons mirin
1 teaspoon xylitol (see note
  page 33)

Put all of the ingredients into a jar and shake well to combine.

Any leftover dressing can be stored in an airtight container in the refrigerator for up to 1 week.

orange and ginger dressing
makes 185 ml (6 fl oz/¾ cup)

60 ml (2 fl oz/¼ cup) coconut oil
  (see note page 36)
1 tablespoon finely grated orange
  zest
60 ml (2 fl oz/¼ cup) freshly
  squeezed orange juice
2 tablespoons shoyu (Japanese
  soy sauce)
1 garlic clove, crushed
2 teaspoons finely grated fresh
  ginger
1 tablespoon xylitol (see note
  page 33)

Put all of the ingredients into a blender and blend until well combined and smooth.

Any leftover dressing can be stored in an airtight container in the refrigerator for up to 2 days.

eggplant yoghurt relish

makes 900 g (2 lb/5 cups)

2 x 150g (5½ oz) eggplants
  (aubergines)
½ teaspoon salt
½ teaspoon turmeric
½ teaspoon chilli powder
100 ml (3½ fl oz) olive oil
2 brown onions, thinly sliced
2 long green chillies, seeded and
  thinly sliced
6 garlic cloves, crushed
2 teaspoons finely grated fresh
  ginger
1 teaspoon dijon mustard
60 ml (2 fl oz/¼ cup) white vinegar
1 teaspoon sugar
125 g (4½ oz/½ cup) plain
  yoghurt

Cut the eggplants into 2 cm (¾ inch) cubes and sprinkle evenly with the combined salt, turmeric and chilli powder.

Heat 1 tablespoon of the oil in a large frying pan over medium–high heat. Add one-quarter of the eggplant and cook for 5 minutes, turning regularly, or until golden brown. Drain on paper towel and place in a large bowl. Repeat with the remaining oil and eggplant until all cooked.

Heat the remaining oil in a frying pan over medium–high heat. Add the onion and cook for 5 minutes, or until starting to soften. Add the chilli, garlic and ginger and cook for a further 2 minutes or until aromatic. Add to the bowl with the eggplant and stir well to combine.

Put the mustard, vinegar, sugar and yoghurt in a bowl and stir well, then add to the eggplant and stir gently until all the ingredients are well combined. Serve immediately.

coconut cream lime dressing

makes 185 ml (6 fl oz/¾ cup)

125 ml (4 fl oz/½ cup) coconut
  cream
freshly squeezed juice of 1 lime
1 tablespoon coconut oil (see
  note page 36)
2 teaspoons xylitol (see note
  page 33)
pinch cayenne pepper

Put all of the ingredients into a jar and shake well to combine.

Any leftover dressing can be stored in an airtight container in the refrigerator for up to 1 week.

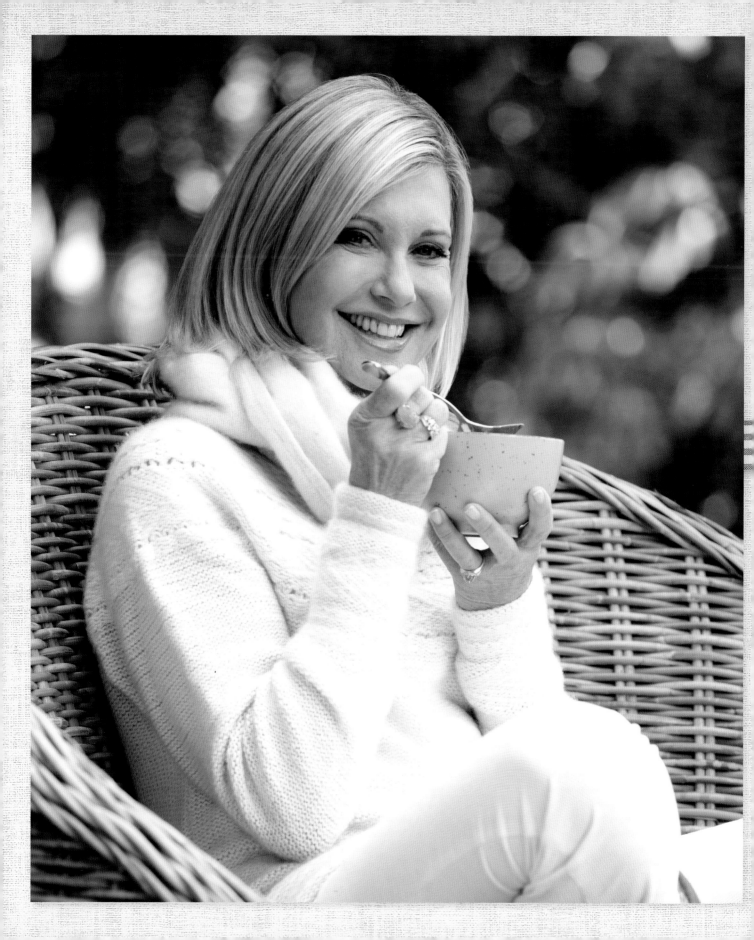

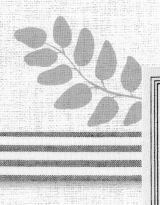

mains

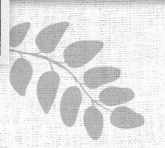

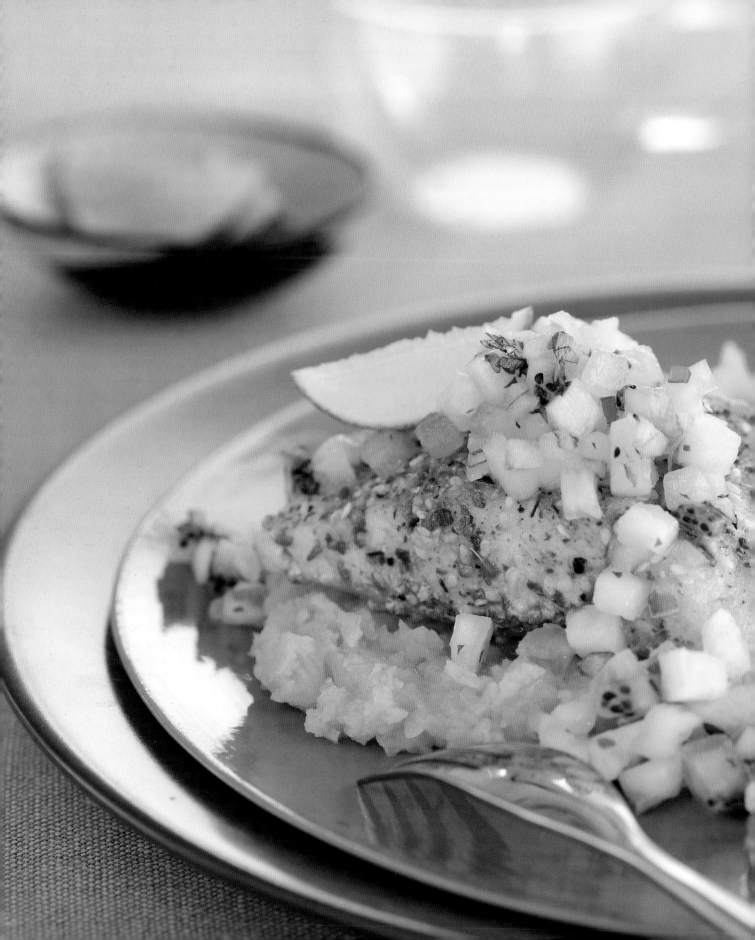

bush-spiced barramundi with sweet potato mash and fruit salsa

serves 4

500 g (1 lb 2 oz) orange sweet
potato, chopped
5 cm (2 inch) piece fresh ginger,
finely grated
50 g (1¾ oz) dukkah (see note)
4 x 165 g (5¾ oz) skinless
barramundi fillets or other firm
white fish fillets
1 tablespoon olive oil
lime wedges, to serve

FRUIT SALSA
½ small red onion, finely chopped
1 kiwi fruit, finely chopped
1 small mango, finely chopped
¼ small pineapple, cored and
finely chopped
2 tablespoons finely chopped
coriander (cilantro) leaves
freshly squeezed juice of 1 lime
2 tablespoons olive oil
1 teaspoon Tabasco sauce, or to
taste

To make the fruit salsa, put all of the ingredients into a bowl and stir to combine. Cover with plastic wrap and refrigerate until needed.

Preheat the oven to 200°C (400°F/Gas 6). Line a baking tray with baking paper.

Cook the sweet potato in a large saucepan of boiling water for 15 minutes, or until tender. Drain well and mash together with the ginger; season with sea salt and freshly ground black pepper. Set aside and keep warm.

Sprinkle the dukkah over the barramundi fillets. Heat the oil in a large frying pan over medium heat and cook the barramundi for about 5 minutes on each side, or until lightly golden on both sides. Transfer the fish to the prepared tray and bake for 8–10 minutes, or until just cooked through.

Divide the sweet potato mash between serving plates, top with the barramundi fillets and spoon some of the fruit salsa over the top. Serve with lime wedges.

Note: Dukkah is a ground nut, seed and spice mixture that is often used as a condiment and flavouring. The version we use at Gaia includes pecans, wattleseeds, hazelnuts, macadamia nuts, sesame seeds, salt, lemon myrtle and coriander. Dukkah is available from some health food stores and speciality grocery stores.

spicy dhal
serves 6–8

500 g (1 lb 2 oz/2 cups) red
   lentils, rinsed
100 g (3½ oz/½ cup) jasmine rice,
   rinsed
200 ml (7 fl oz) coconut milk
1 carrot, finely diced
¼ small cauliflower, cut into
   small florets
1 cinnamon stick
1 bay leaf
3 teaspoons yellow curry paste
¼ teaspoon green curry paste
1 teaspoon sea salt
3 teaspoons boiling water
50 g (1¾ oz) baby spinach leaves
80 g (2¾ oz/½ cup) frozen peas
1 teaspoon olive oil
½ teaspoon fennel seeds
½ teaspoon cumin seeds
½ teaspoon ground turmeric
½ teaspoon ground coriander
½ teaspoon vegetable stock
   (bouillon) powder
½ teaspoon xylitol (see note
   page 33)
½ teaspoon freshly ground black
   pepper
Greek-style yoghurt, to serve

Put the lentils, rice and 1 litre (35 fl oz/4 cups) water in
a large saucepan over high heat. Bring to the boil, then
reduce the heat to medium–low, add the coconut milk,
carrot, cauliflower, cinnamon stick and bay leaf and simmer,
uncovered, for 15 minutes.

Put the yellow and green curry pastes in a small bowl with
½ teaspoon of the sea salt and the boiling water and stir
well to combine. Add to the lentil mixture and cook, stirring
occasionally, for a further 15 minutes, or until the lentils are
tender. Stir in the spinach and peas and cook for 3 minutes,
or until the spinach has wilted and is bright green. Discard
the cinnamon stick and bay leaf.

Meanwhile, heat the olive oil in a small frying pan over high
heat. Add the fennel seeds, cumin seeds, turmeric and
coriander and cook for 30 seconds, or until aromatic. Transfer
to a bowl and add the stock powder, xylitol, remaining salt
and the pepper and stir to combine.

Serve the warm dhal with the seeds and spices sprinkled over
the top and the yoghurt on the side.

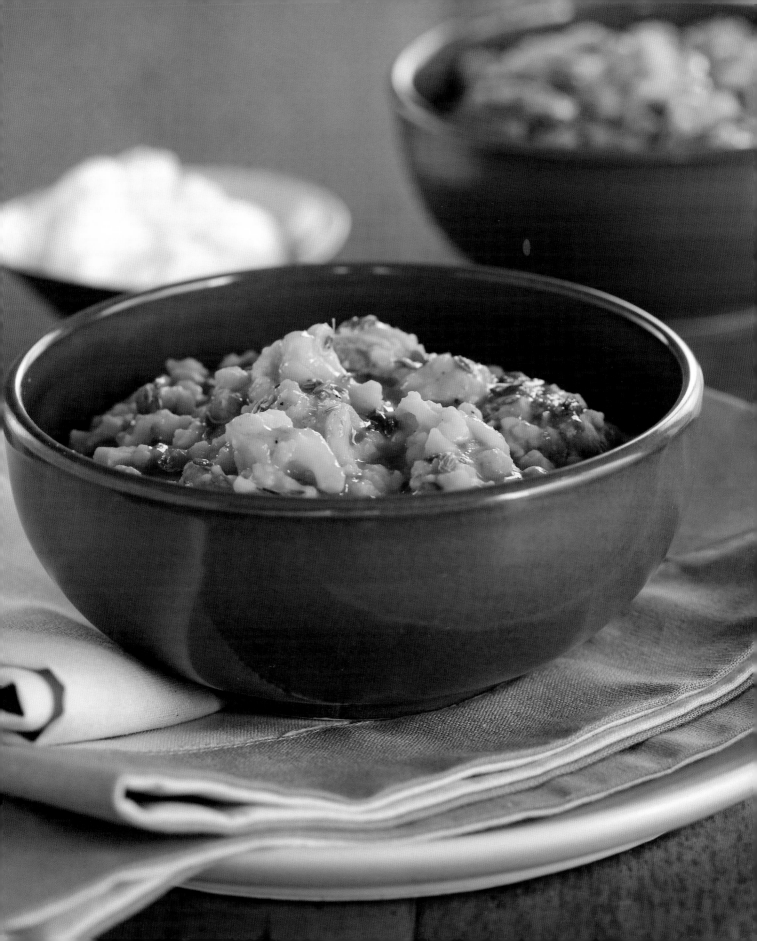

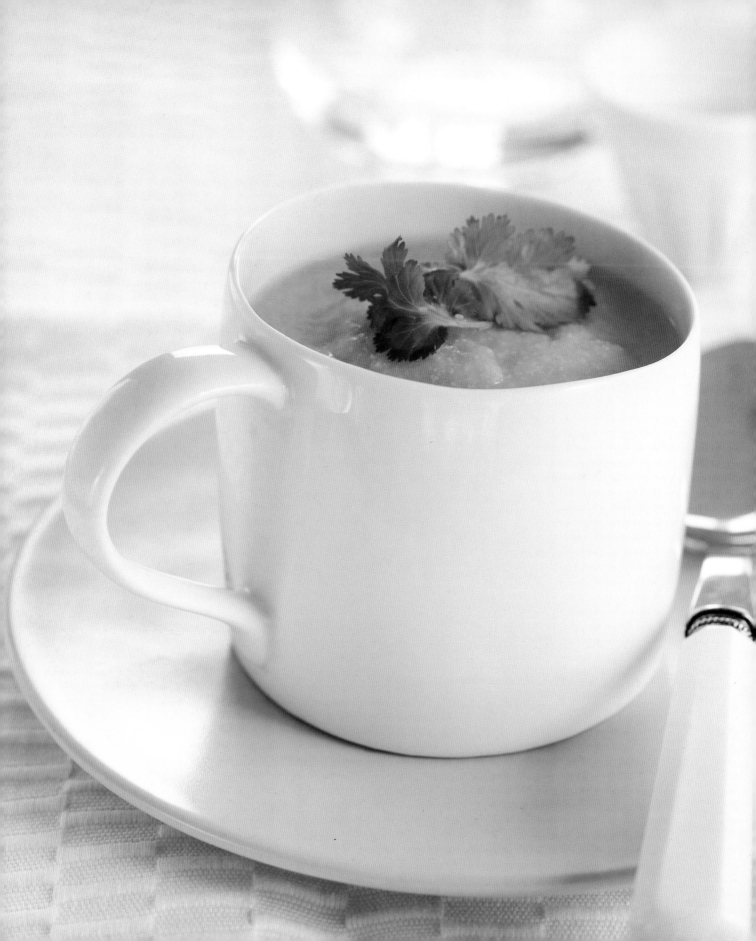

carrot cashew soup

serves 4–6

155 g (5½ oz/1 cup) cashew nuts
2 tablespoons macadamia oil
2 brown onions, coarsely chopped
8 cm (3¼ inch) piece fresh ginger,
    finely chopped
1 kg (2 lb 4 oz) carrots, coarsely
    chopped
pinch cayenne pepper, or to taste
fresh coriander (cilantro) leaves,
    to serve

Rinse the cashews under cold running water and drain. Place in a bowl and pour over enough water to cover, then set aside and soak overnight. Drain well.

Heat the macadamia oil in a large saucepan over medium–high heat. Add the onion and ginger and cook for about 5 minutes, or until the onion softens. Add the cashews, carrot and 1.5 litres (52 fl oz/6 cups) water. Bring to the boil, then reduce the heat to medium–low and simmer, uncovered, for about 15 minutes, or until the carrot is tender. Stir in the cayenne pepper, then remove from the heat and allow to cool slightly.

Transfer the soup to a food processor or blender and process, in batches, until smooth. Return the soup to the pan over medium heat until heated through. Serve topped with the coriander leaves.

Olivia's lemon chicken
serves 4–6

1.2 kg (2 lb 10 oz) organic chicken
1 large lemon
2 tablespoons olive oil or melted
   butter
roasted orange sweet potato,
   to serve
steamed broccoli or green salad,
   to serve

Preheat the oven to 200°C (400°F/Gas 4). Lightly grease a roasting tin and place a wire rack in the base of the tin.

Trim any excess fat from the chicken and discard the neck. Rinse the chicken (including the cavity) under cold running water and pat dry with paper towel. Season the cavity with sea salt and freshly ground black pepper.

Using a fork or metal skewer, prick the lemon all over and place inside the chicken cavity. Rub the oil all over the outside of the chicken and season well. Roast the chicken for 45 minutes–1 hour, or until the juices run clear when the thigh is pierced with a skewer. Remove from the oven and allow to rest, covered, for 10 minutes before serving.

Serve the roast chicken with orange sweet potato, the steamed broccoli or a green salad.

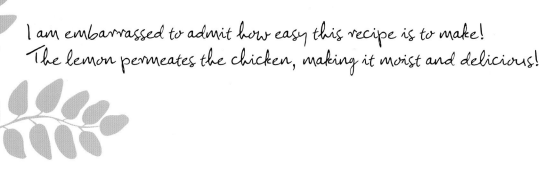

I am embarrassed to admit how easy this recipe is to make! The lemon permeates the chicken, making it moist and delicious!

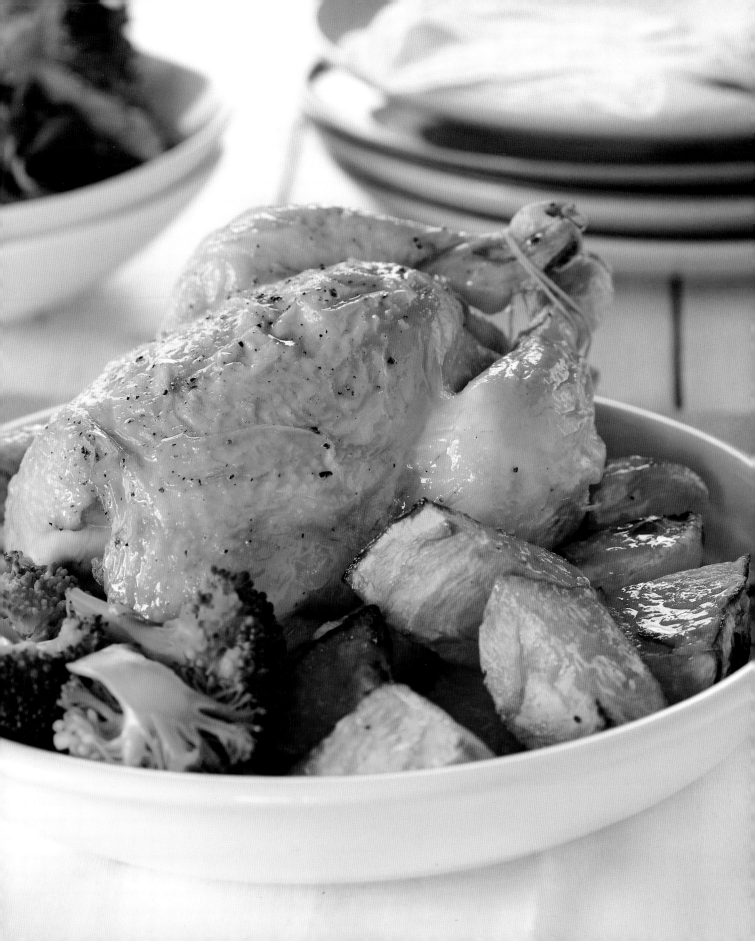

mexican chilli beef tacos

serves 6

2 brown onions, finely chopped

1 garlic clove, crushed

500 g (1 lb 2 oz) lean minced (ground) beef

2 beef stock (bouillon) cubes

2 tablespoons tomato paste (concentrated purée)

2 teaspoons chilli powder

½ teaspoon ground cumin

½ teaspoon ground coriander

½ teaspoon dried oregano

400 g (14 oz) tin red kidney beans, drained

12 taco shells

shredded lettuce, to serve

grated low-fat cheddar cheese, to serve

finely chopped tomatoes, to serve

diced avocado, to serve

Heat 2 tablespoons water in a large frying pan over medium heat. Add the onion and garlic and cook for 4 minutes, or until the onion softens. Add the beef, increase the heat to medium–high and cook for 5 minutes, breaking up any large lumps of meat with a spoon, until the mince has browned. Add the stock cubes, tomato paste, chilli powder, cumin, coriander, oregano and 500 ml (17 fl oz/2 cups) water and stir until well combined. Bring to the boil over high heat, then reduce the heat to low and simmer for 30 minutes, or until thickened.

Add the kidney beans and stir to combine. Bring the mixture to the boil, then remove from the heat and keep warm.

Heat the taco shells following the packet directions. Place on a platter with the lettuce, cheese, tomato and avocado. Serve the chilli beef in a bowl and allow guests to assemble their own tacos.

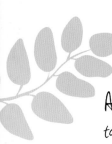

Always a favourite. Try flour tortillas or lavash instead of tacos to reduce the fat and kilojoule count.

ocean trout on pea and yoghurt mash

serves 4

450 g (1 lb/3 cups) fresh or frozen
   green peas
1 large brown onion, chopped
435 g (15¼ oz/1¾ cups) Greek-
   style yoghurt
4 x 165 g (5¾ oz) skinless,
   boneless ocean trout or salmon
   fillets
1 tablespoon olive oil
1 tablespoon chopped flat-leaf
   (Italian) parsley
1 tablespoon snipped chives
1 tablespoon chopped mint

Cook the peas and onion in a saucepan of boiling water for
2–4 minutes, or until tender. Use a fork to mash together the
peas and onion, then stir through 185 g (6½ oz/¾ cup) of the
yoghurt. Set aside and keep warm until ready to serve.

Brush the fish lightly on both sides with the oil and cook on
a preheated chargrill plate or frying pan over medium–high
heat for 3 minutes on each side, or until almost cooked
through.

Serve the fish with the pea and yoghurt mash on the side
and a dollop of the remaining yoghurt on top. Sprinkle
with the combined herbs and season with freshly ground
black pepper.

This is a healthy meal option that's quick to make but makes an impact at a dinner party as well.

chickpea patties
makes 8 (serves 4)

600 g (1 lb 5 oz) all-purpose
   potatoes
2 x 400 g (14 oz) tins chickpeas,
   rinsed and drained
1 carrot, grated
1 brown onion, finely chopped
1 garlic clove, crushed
¼ cup coriander (cilantro) leaves,
   finely chopped
2 teaspoons vegetable stock
   (bouillon) powder
½ teaspoon sea salt
1 tablespoon sunflower seeds,
   ground
2 tablespoons tahini
1 free-range egg
35 g (1¼ oz/¼ cup) fine polenta
olive oil, for frying

Preheat the oven to 200°C (400°F/Gas 6). Line a baking tray with baking paper.

Peel and slice the potatoes. Cook them in a saucepan of boiling water for 15 minutes, or until very tender. Drain well. Mash in a large bowl until smooth and then allow to cool.

Add the chickpeas, carrot, onion, garlic, coriander, stock powder, salt, ground sunflower seeds and tahini to the mashed potato. Mash the ingredients together until well combined. Add the egg and stir well to combine.

Take half a cup of mixture at a time and shape into patties. Roll the patties in the polenta to coat lightly and set aside on the prepared tray.

Heat a little olive oil in a large frying pan over medium–high heat. Cook the patties, in batches, for about 2 minutes on each side, or until golden brown. Return the patties to the prepared tray and bake in the oven for about 20 minutes, or until heated through. Serve with your favourite salad and dressing (see pages 80–107).

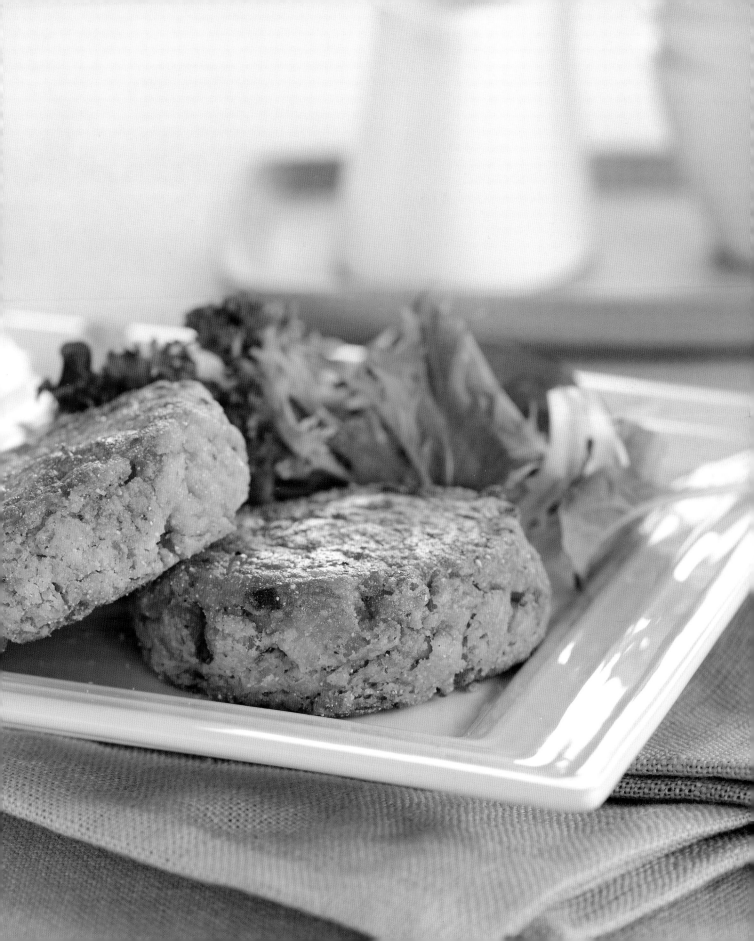

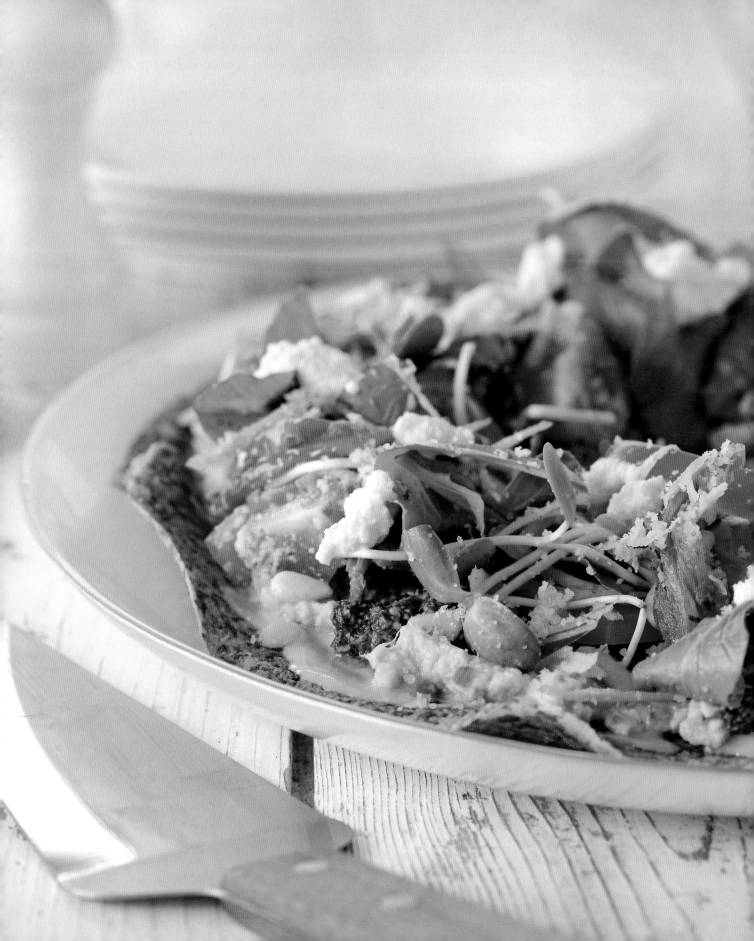

pizza italiano
serves 2

30 g (1 oz) rocket (arugula) leaves

1 small carrot, coarsely grated

2 tablespoons semi-dried
(sun-blushed) tomatoes

¼ red onion, thinly sliced

¼ red capsicum (pepper), seeded,
membrane removed and cut
into thin strips

⅓ cup sprouted sunflower seeds
(see pages 14–15)

1 tablespoon basil leaves, torn

2 teaspoons pine nuts

3 cherry tomatoes, quartered

1–2 tablespoons vegan parmesan
cheese (see page 76)

1 pizza base (see page 70)

2 tablespoons tahini

½ quantity avocado salsa (see
page 75)

2 tablespoons pesto (see
page 71)

1 roma (plum) tomato, thinly
sliced

vegan cream cheese (see
page 76), to serve

Put the rocket, carrot, semi-dried tomatoes, onion, capsicum, sunflower sprouts, basil, pine nuts, cherry tomato and vegan parmesan cheese into a large bowl and toss to combine.

Spread the pizza base with tahini, avocado salsa and pesto. Top with tomato slices and the combined vegetables. Serve with the vegan cream cheese spooned over the top.

mushroom soup with lemon and thyme

serves 4

1 tablespoon extra virgin olive oil

1 large brown onion, coarsely
   chopped

2 garlic cloves, crushed

300 g (10½ oz) mixed field
   mushrooms, coarsely chopped

100 ml (3½ fl oz) dry white wine

2 all-purpose potatoes, chopped

1 litre (35 fl oz/4 cups) vegetable
   stock

2 teaspoons thyme leaves,
   plus extra sprigs (optional),
   to garnish

1–2 teaspoons finely grated
   lemon zest

1 bay leaf

Heat the olive oil in a large saucepan over high heat. Add the onion, garlic and mushrooms and cook for about 5 minutes, or until the onion softens. Add the wine and simmer until it has almost evaporated.

Add the potato, stock, thyme, lemon zest and bay leaf and bring to the boil. Reduce the heat to medium–low and simmer, uncovered, for 15 minutes, or until the potato is tender. Remove from the heat and allow to cool slightly. Discard the bay leaf.

Transfer the soup to a food processor or blender, in batches, and process until smooth. Return the soup to the pan over medium heat until warm. Serve immediately, garnished with thyme sprigs, if desired.

This soup is a beautiful combination of mushrooms, lemon and thyme. The soup has an amazing array of earthy flavours and is a favourite at Gaia. We use only organic ingredients when making this delicious soup.

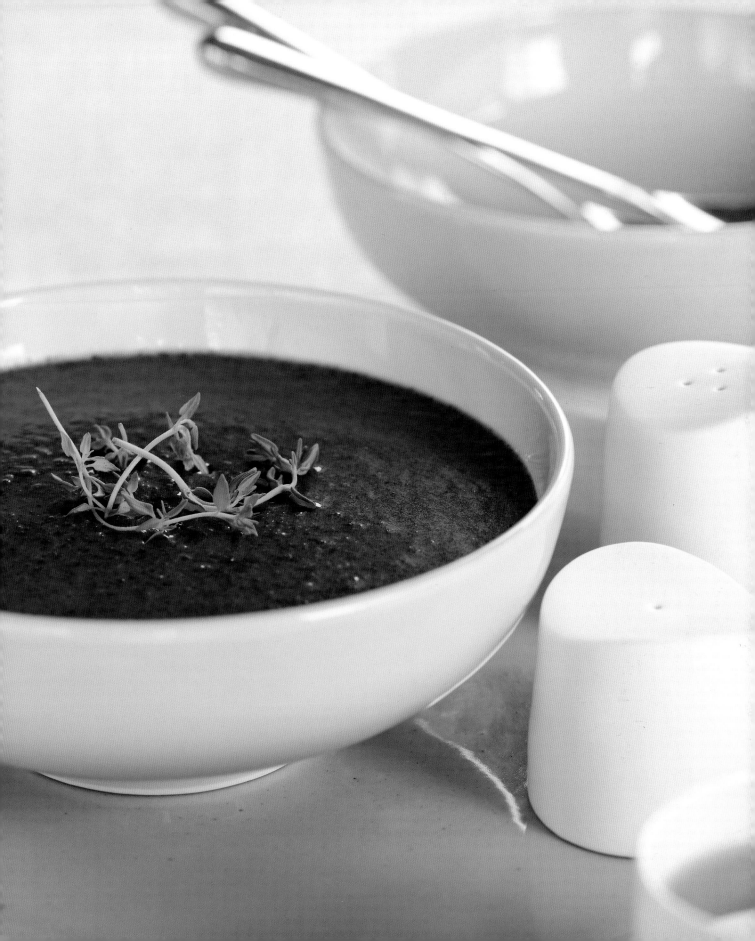

spiced beef rosemary skewers with yoghurt sauce

serves 4–6

10 woody rosemary stems with
   leaves attached (about
   15 cm/6 inches long)
1 kg (2 lb 4 oz) lean rump steak,
   coarsely ground
½ teaspoon freshly grated
   nutmeg
½ teaspoon ground cloves
½ teaspoon ground cinnamon
olive oil, for cooking

YOGHURT SAUCE
250 g (9 oz/1 cup) Greek-style
   yoghurt
2 garlic cloves, crushed
freshly squeezed juice of 1 lemon

Soak the rosemary stems in water for 5 minutes. Drain well and set aside.

To make the yoghurt sauce, put the yoghurt, garlic and lemon juice into a bowl and stir well to combine. Cover with plastic wrap and refrigerate until needed.

Put the beef, nutmeg, cloves and cinnamon into a bowl and use your hands to mix well until evenly combined. With well-oiled hands, take one-third of a cup of the mixture at a time and press it around a rosemary stem.

Preheat a chargrill plate or barbecue grill to medium–high. Lightly brush with oil and cook the skewers for 5–8 minutes, turning occasionally, until just cooked through. Serve immediately with a dollop of the yoghurt sauce on top.

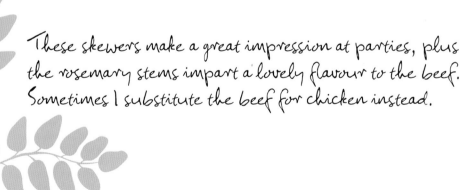

These skewers make a great impression at parties, plus the rosemary stems impart a lovely flavour to the beef. Sometimes I substitute the beef for chicken instead.

thai barbecue chicken
serves 4

4 chicken breast fillets, trimmed
steamed jasmine rice, to serve
olive oil spray, for cooking

MARINADE
1 bunch coriander (cilantro)
1–2 lemongrass stems, white part
  only, chopped
5 garlic cloves
1 teaspoon ground turmeric
1 teaspoon coriander seeds
1½ teaspoons black peppercorns
1½ teaspoons soft brown sugar
250 g (9 oz/1 cup) plain yoghurt

To make the marinade, trim the roots from the coriander and rinse well. Reserve the leaves and stems for another use. Put the coriander roots, lemongrass, garlic, turmeric, coriander seeds, peppercorns and sugar in a food processor with 2 tablespoons of the yoghurt and process until smooth. Add the remaining yoghurt and process until just combined.

Place the chicken in a large shallow bowl, pour over the marinade and turn to coat, making sure the chicken is well coated. Cover with plastic wrap and refrigerate for at least 2 hours.

Preheat a chargrill plate to medium–high. Lightly oil the plate and cook the chicken for 3–4 minutes on each side, or until just cooked through. Serve immediately with steamed rice.

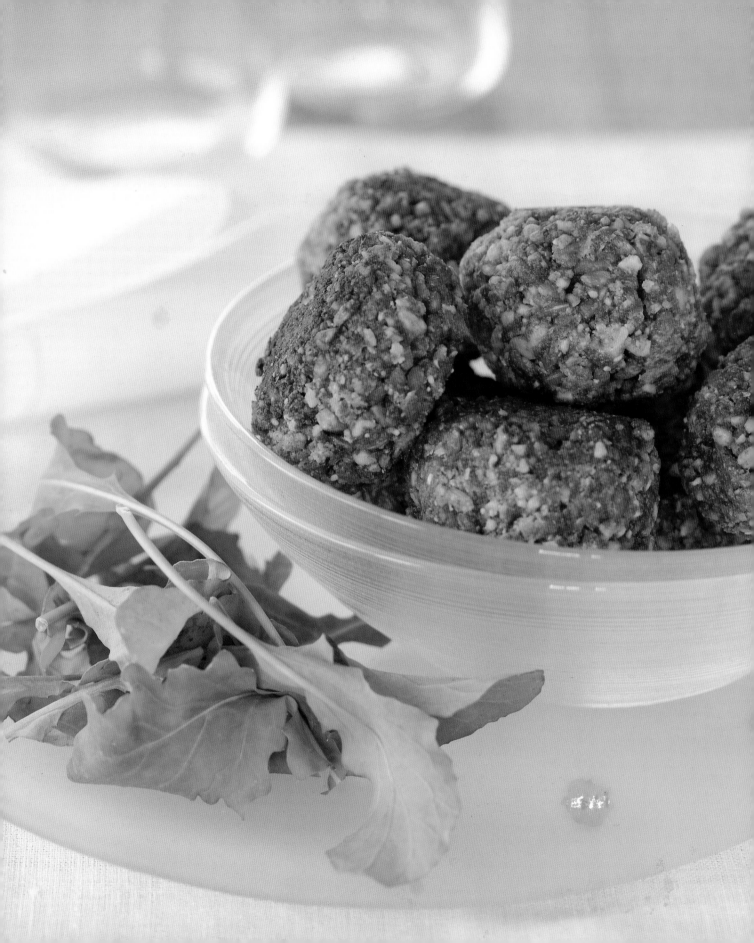

walnut patties

serves 4

115 g (4 oz/1 cup) ground walnuts

185 g (6½ oz/1 cup) cooked
brown rice

40 g (1½ oz/¼ cup) spelt flour

80 g (2¾ oz/1 cup) fresh
breadcrumbs

½ teaspoon sea salt

½ teaspoon dried sage

1 garlic clove, crushed

2 teaspoons vegetable stock
(bouillon) powder

3 tablespoons almond butter
(see note)

2 tablespoons soy sauce

olive oil, for frying

Preheat the oven to 200°C (400°F/Gas 6). Line a baking tray with baking paper.

Put the ground walnuts, cooked rice, flour, breadcrumbs, salt, sage, garlic, stock powder, almond butter and soy sauce into a large bowl and stir well to combine. Set aside for about 15 minutes.

Take one-quarter of a cup of mixture at a time and shape it into patties. Repeat to make 10 patties in total.

Heat a little olive oil in a large frying pan over medium–high heat. Cook the patties, in batches, for 2 minutes on each side, or until golden brown. Transfer to the prepared tray and bake for about 10 minutes, or until heated through.

Serve the walnut patties with your favourite salad and dressing (see pages 80–107).

Note: Almond butter is made from almonds that are blended to make a paste. It is available from selected supermarkets and health food stores.

chickpea casserole
serves 6–8

1 tablespoon olive oil

1 large brown onion, diced

1 red capsicum (pepper), seeded, membrane removed and diced

2 garlic cloves, crushed

1 teaspoon dried oregano

400 g (14 oz/2 cups) chopped tomatoes

1 tablespoon tomato paste (concentrated purée)

2 x 400 g (14 oz) tins chickpeas, rinsed and drained

1 carrot, diced

2 large potatoes, diced

1 teaspoon sea salt

1 tablespoon vegetable stock (bouillon) powder

2 tablespoons chopped flat-leaf (Italian) parsley

Heat the oil in a large saucepan over medium–high heat. Add the onion, capsicum, garlic and oregano and cook for about 5 minutes, stirring often, until the onion softens.

Add the tomato, tomato paste, chickpeas, carrot, potato, salt, stock powder and enough water to just cover the vegetables. Bring to the boil, then reduce the heat to medium–low and simmer, partially covered, for 25–30 minutes. Remove from the heat, stir in the parsley and serve immediately.

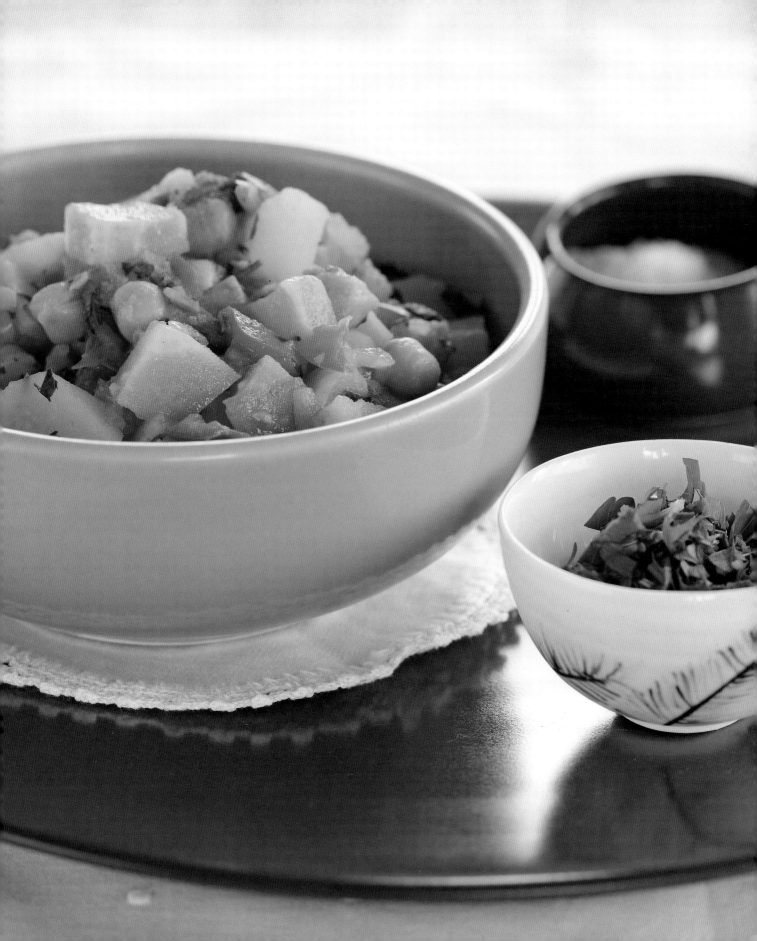

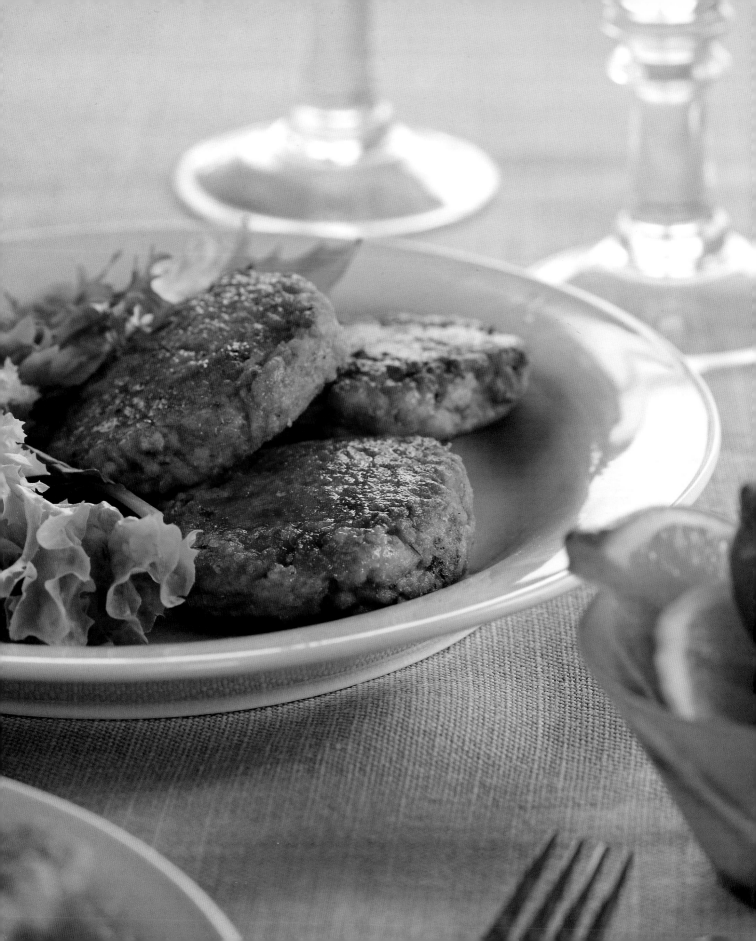

vegie patties
serves 6 (makes about 12)

400 g (14 oz) all-purpose
  potatoes, coarsely grated
1 large zucchini (courgette),
  coarsely grated
1 large onion, coarsely grated
400 g (14 oz) orange sweet
  potato, peeled and coarsely
  grated
1 carrot, coarsely grated
1 garlic clove, crushed
2 teaspoons finely grated fresh
  ginger
1 cup flat-leaf (Italian) parsley,
  finely chopped
½ teaspoon ground coriander
½ teaspoon dried rosemary
½ teaspoon dried oregano
½ teaspoon sea salt
3 free-range eggs, lightly beaten
120 g (4¼ oz/¾ cup) spelt flour
olive oil, for cooking

Preheat the oven to 200°C (400°F/Gas 6). Line a baking tray with baking paper.

Put the potato, zucchini and onion in a colander and use your hands to squeeze out as much moisture as possible. Put these into a large bowl and add the sweet potato, carrot, garlic, ginger, parsley, coriander, rosemary, oregano, salt, egg and 80 g (2¾ oz/½ cup) of the flour and stir until well combined. Cover and set aside for 15 minutes.

Take one-quarter of a cup of the mixture at a time and push the mixture into a patty shape. Roll in the remaining flour to coat both sides. Repeat with the remaining mixture to make about 12 in total.

Heat a little olive oil in a large frying pan over medium–high heat. Cook the patties, in batches, for 3–4 minutes on each side, or until golden brown. Transfer to the prepared tray and bake for about 20 minutes, or until cooked through. Serve the fritters with your favourite salad and dressing (see pages 80–107).

Note: This mixture may be a little wet and therefore a little difficult to shape, however the moisture will add to the lightness of these patties.

lentil and spinach casserole

serves 6–8

1 tablespoon olive oil

1 brown onion, finely chopped

2 garlic cloves, crushed

1 red capsicum (pepper), seeded, membrane removed and diced

1 teaspoon sea salt

2 teaspoons ground coriander

¼ teaspoon asafoetida powder (see note)

¼ teaspoon cayenne pepper

1 tablespoon vegetable stock (bouillon) powder

4 ripe tomatoes, chopped

1 tablespoon tomato paste (concentrated purée)

400 g (14 oz) tin brown lentils, rinsed and drained

1 carrot, diced

2 large all-purpose potatoes, diced

juice of ½ lemon

1 teaspoon xylitol (see note page 33)

2 tablespoons chopped flat-leaf (Italian) parsley

5 spinach leaves, shredded

steamed rice or chapatti (see page 67), to serve

Heat the oil in a large, heavy-based saucepan over medium–high heat. Add the onion, garlic and capsicum and cook for about 5 minutes, stirring often, until the onion softens. Add the salt, coriander, asafoetida powder, cayenne pepper and stock powder and cook, stirring, for 1 minute, or until aromatic.

Add the tomato, tomato paste, lentils, carrot, potato, lemon juice, xylitol and enough water to just cover the vegetables. Bring to the boil, then reduce the heat to medium–low and simmer, covered, for 25–30 minutes. Remove from the heat and stir in the parsley and spinach leaves. Serve with steamed rice or chapatti.

Note: Asafoetida powder is used widely in Indian cooking and is a powdered flavouring obtained from a large, fennel-like plant. Because of its pungency, it is always used in small quantities. It is available from Indian grocery stores and some health food stores.

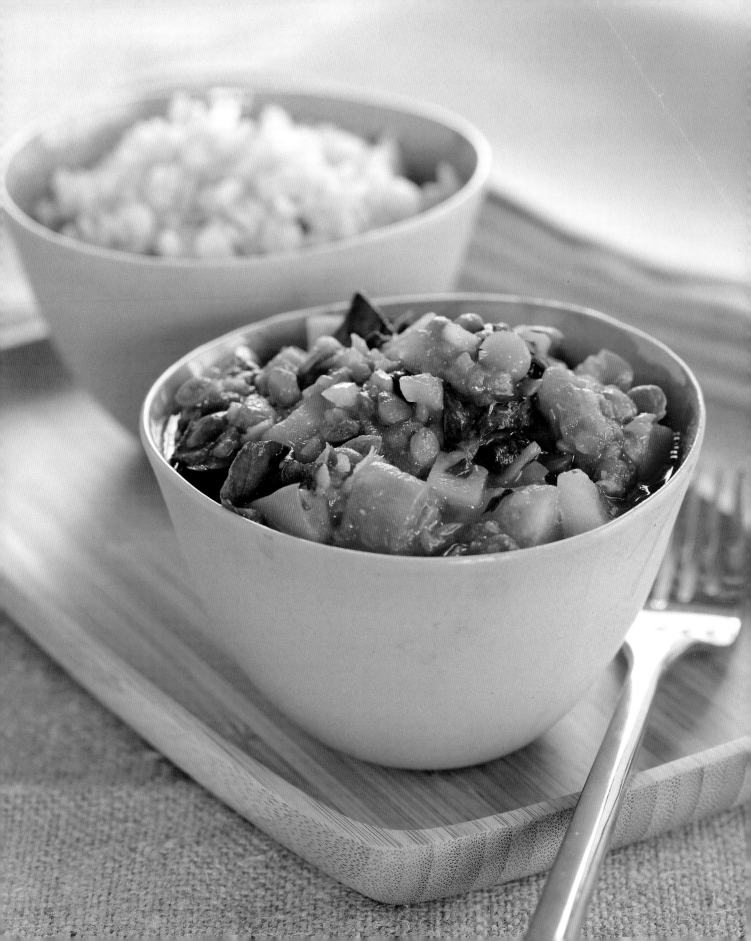

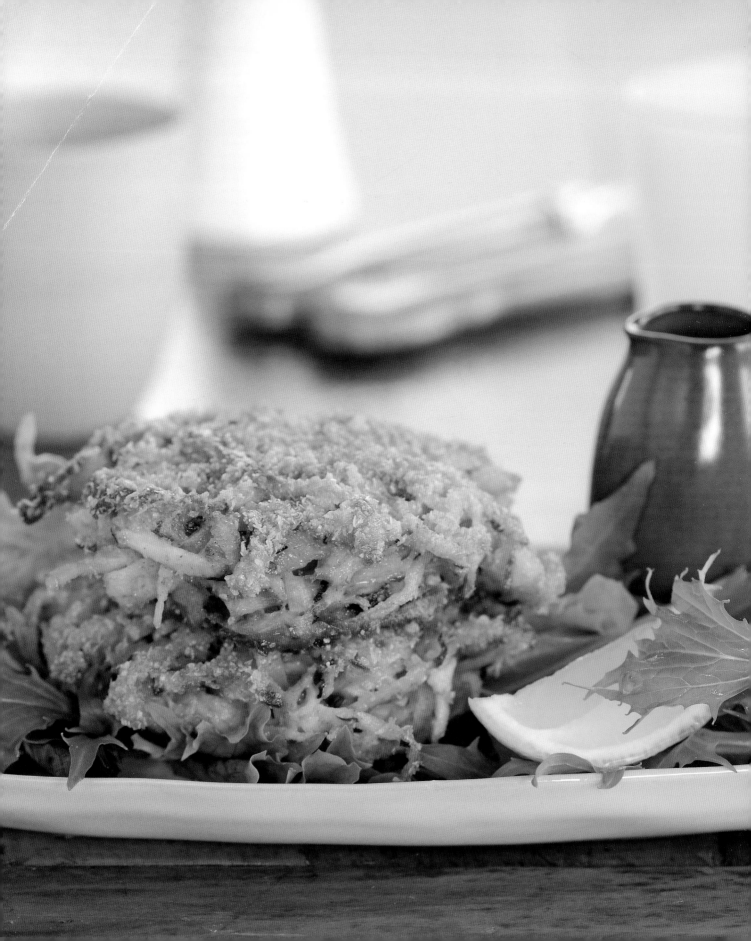

zucchini and carrot patties

serves 4

1 large zucchini (courgette),
   grated
450 g (1 lb/3 cups) grated carrot
120 g (4¼ oz/¾ cup) spelt flour
1 brown onion, finely chopped
1 garlic clove, crushed
¼ cup flat-leaf (Italian) parsley,
   finely chopped
¼ teaspoon dried rosemary
¼ teaspoon kelp powder
   (see note)
½ teaspoon sea salt
3 free-range eggs, lightly beaten
45 g (1¾ oz/½ cup) wheat germ
coconut oil (see note page 36),
   for frying

Preheat the oven to 200°C (400°F/Gas 6). Line a baking tray with baking paper.

Put the zucchini, carrot, flour, onion, garlic, parsley, rosemary, kelp powder, salt and egg into a large bowl and stir well until completely combined.

Take half a cup of mixture at a time and shape into a large patty. Roll in the wheat germ to coat on both sides. Repeat with the remaining mixture to make 10 patties in total.

Heat a little coconut oil in a large frying pan over medium–low heat. Cook the patties, in batches, for 2 minutes on each side, or until browned all over. Transfer to the prepared tray and bake for about 10 minutes, or until cooked through. Serve the zucchini and carrot patties with your favourite salad and dressing (see pages 80–107).

Note: Kelp is a sea vegetable packed with nutrients, particularly iodine. Iodine helps the thyroid to function correctly and is also known to support the immune system. Kelp powder is available from health food stores and some chemists.

haricot bean and rice bake

serves 6

1 tablespoon coconut oil (see
    note page 36)
1 large brown onion, finely
    chopped
1 garlic clove, crushed
4 large ripe tomatoes, chopped
2 x 400 g (14 oz) tins haricot
    beans, rinsed and drained
185 g (6½ oz/1 cup) cooked
    brown rice
1 cup flat-leaf (Italian) parsley,
    finely chopped
1 vegetarian stock (bouillon) cube
1 teaspoon sea salt
1 teaspoon thyme leaves
cayenne pepper, to taste
80 g (2¾ oz/1 cup) fresh
    breadcrumbs
2 tablespoons ground almonds

Preheat the oven to 180°C (350°F/Gas 4). Lightly grease a
1.5 litre (52 fl oz/6 cup) capacity baking dish.

Heat the coconut oil in a large saucepan over high heat. Add
the onion and garlic and cook for about 5 minutes, or until
the onion softens. Add the tomato, beans, rice, parsley, stock
cube, salt, thyme and 125 ml (4 fl oz/½ cup) water. Cook for
15–20 minutes, stirring occasionally, or until thickened slightly.
Season to taste with the cayenne pepper.

Transfer the bean mixture to the prepared dish and sprinkle
with the combined breadcrumbs and ground almonds. Bake
for about 30 minutes, or until golden. Remove from the oven
and allow to stand for 10 minutes before serving.

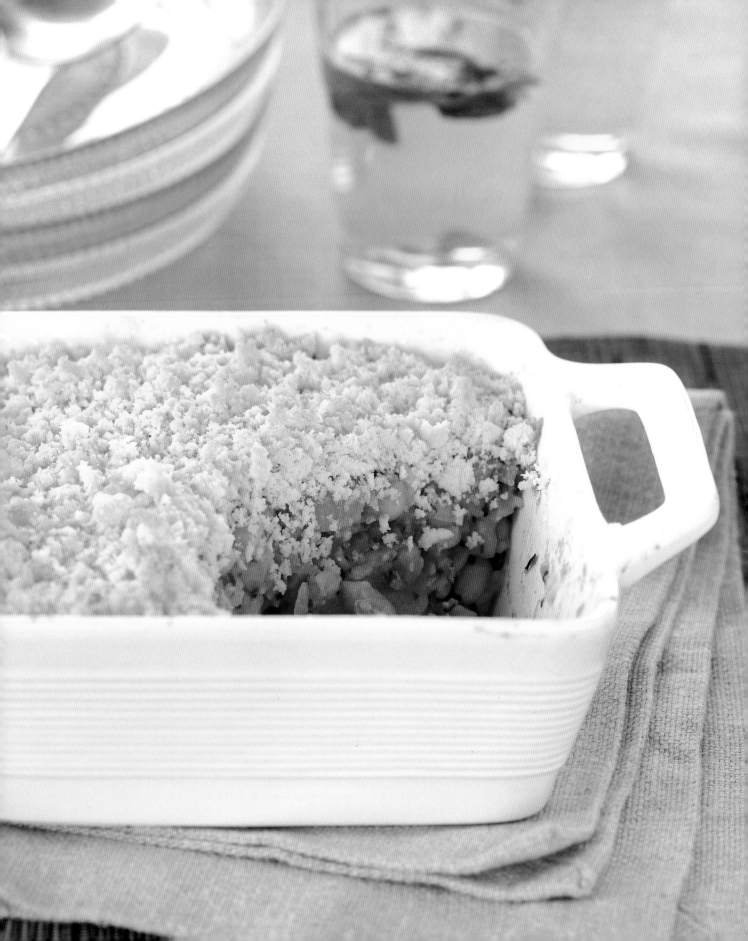

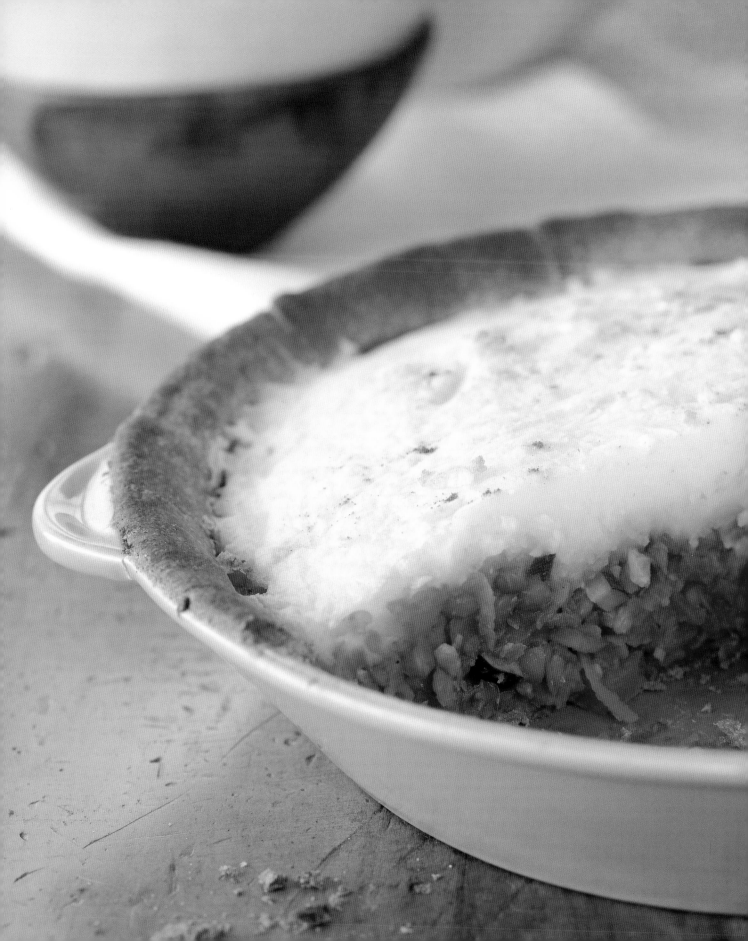

potato and lentil pie

serves 8

SPELT PASTRY

120 g (4¼ oz/¾ cup) spelt flour
110 g (3¾ oz/¾ cup) self-raising
   spelt flour
½ teaspoon salt
2 tablespoons olive oil

LENTIL FILLING

1 tablespoon olive oil
1 small brown onion, finely chopped
2 garlic cloves, crushed
½ red capsicum (pepper), seeded,
   membrane removed and finely
   chopped
4 button mushrooms, finely chopped
400 g (14 oz) tin chopped tomatoes
1 tablespoon tomato paste
   (concentrated purée)
1 small carrot, grated
1 small zucchini (courgette), diced
1 tablespoon vegetable stock
   (bouillon) powder
400 g (14 oz) tin brown lentils,
   rinsed and drained
95 g (3¼ oz/½ cup) cooked brown
   rice
¼ cup chopped flat-leaf (Italian)
   parsley

POTATO TOPPING

3 large all-purpose potatoes, diced
½ teaspoon sea salt
2 tablespoons oat milk
1 tablespoon olive oil
pinch paprika

Grease a 23 cm (9 inch) round pie dish, about 4 cm
(1½ inches) deep.

To make the spelt pastry, sift both of the flours and salt
together into a large bowl. Using your fingers, rub the oil
into the flour until the mixture resembles fine breadcrumbs.
Gradually stir in 80 ml (2½ fl oz/⅓ cup) boiling water until
the mixture forms a dough. Turn out onto a lightly floured
surface and knead the dough gently until smooth. Divide into
two portions and roll out one portion between two sheets of
baking paper to make a circle with a 25 cm (10 inch) diameter,
about 3 mm (⅛ inch) thick. Carefully lower the pastry into the
dish, trimming any excess. Set aside.

To make the lentil filling, heat the oil in a large saucepan
over medium–high heat. Add the onion, garlic and capsicum
and cook for about 5 minutes, stirring often, until the onion
softens. Add the mushroom and cook for 5 minutes, or until
softened. Add the tomatoes, tomato paste and 185 ml
(6 fl oz/¾ cup) water. Bring to the boil. Add the carrot,
zucchini, stock powder, lentils and rice. Reduce the heat to
medium–low and simmer, uncovered, for 10 minutes, or until
the vegetables are tender and the mixture has thickened. Stir
in the parsley and set aside to cool.

Preheat the oven to 200°C (400°F/Gas 6).

To make the potato topping, cook the potato in a large
saucepan of boiling water for 15 minutes, or until very tender.
Drain well and mash together with the salt, oat milk and oil
until well combined and smooth.

Spoon the cooled lentil filling over the pastry in the dish
and layer the mashed potato over the top. Sprinkle with the
paprika and bake for about 40 minutes, or until the topping
is lightly browned. Remove from the oven and allow to stand
for 10 minutes before cutting into slices and serving.

ocean trout with cauliflower purée and lime balsamic dressing

serves 4

4 x 165 g (5¾ oz) skinless ocean trout fillets

185 ml (6 fl oz/¾ cup) freshly squeezed orange juice

⅓ cup chopped dill

1 small cauliflower, cut into small florets

125 ml (4 fl oz/½ cup) macadamia oil

4 bok choy (pak choy), trimmed and halved, to serve

LIME BALSAMIC DRESSING

55 ml (1¾ fl oz) macadamia oil

55 ml (1¾ fl oz) freshly squeezed lime juice

2 tablespoons white balsamic vinegar

1 teaspoon dijon mustard

Put the trout, orange juice and dill in a glass or ceramic dish and turn the fillets to coat in the marinade. Cover with plastic wrap and refrigerate for 3 hours.

To make the lime balsamic dressing, put the macadamia oil, lime juice, vinegar and mustard in a small bowl and whisk well until combined. Set aside until needed.

Preheat the oven to 200°C (400°F/Gas 6). Line a baking tray with baking paper.

Cook the cauliflower in a large saucepan of boiling water for 15–20 minutes, or until very tender. Drain well, then transfer to a food processor with 100 ml (3½ fl oz) of the macadamia oil and process until smooth. Cover to keep warm.

Remove the fillets from the marinade and pat dry with paper towel. Heat the remaining macadamia oil in a large frying pan and cook the trout for 4 minutes on each side, or until browned. Transfer to the prepared tray and bake for 8–10 minutes, or until cooked to your liking.

Meanwhile, bring a large saucepan of water to the boil. Add the bok choy and blanch for 30 seconds, or until tender. Drain well.

Divide the cauliflower purée between serving plates, top with the trout and drizzle the lime balsamic dressing over the top. Serve with the blanched bok choy alongside.

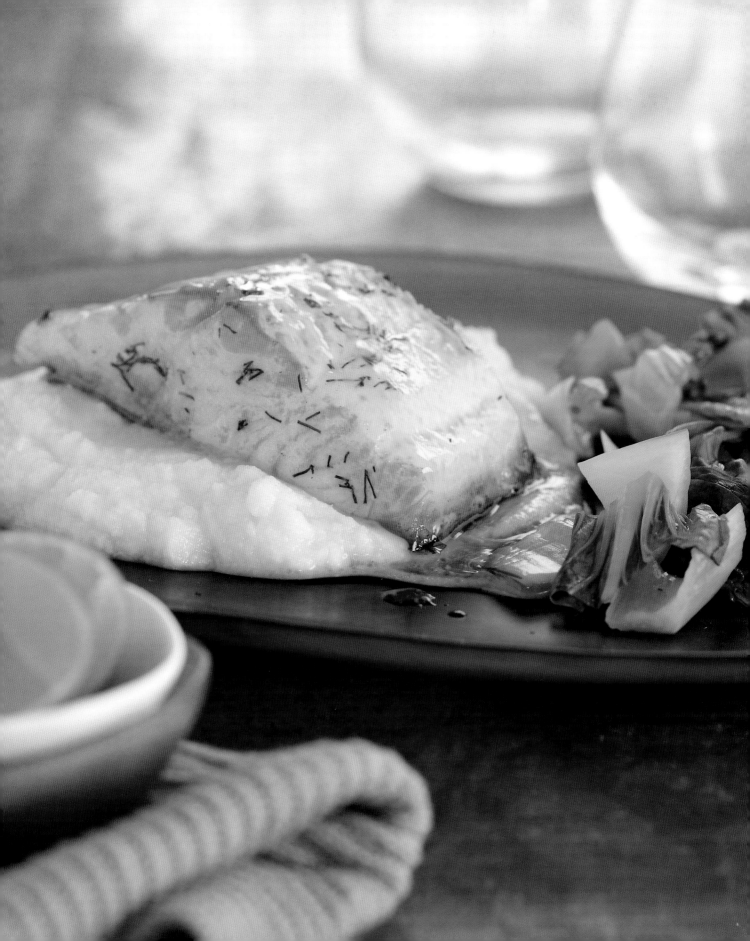

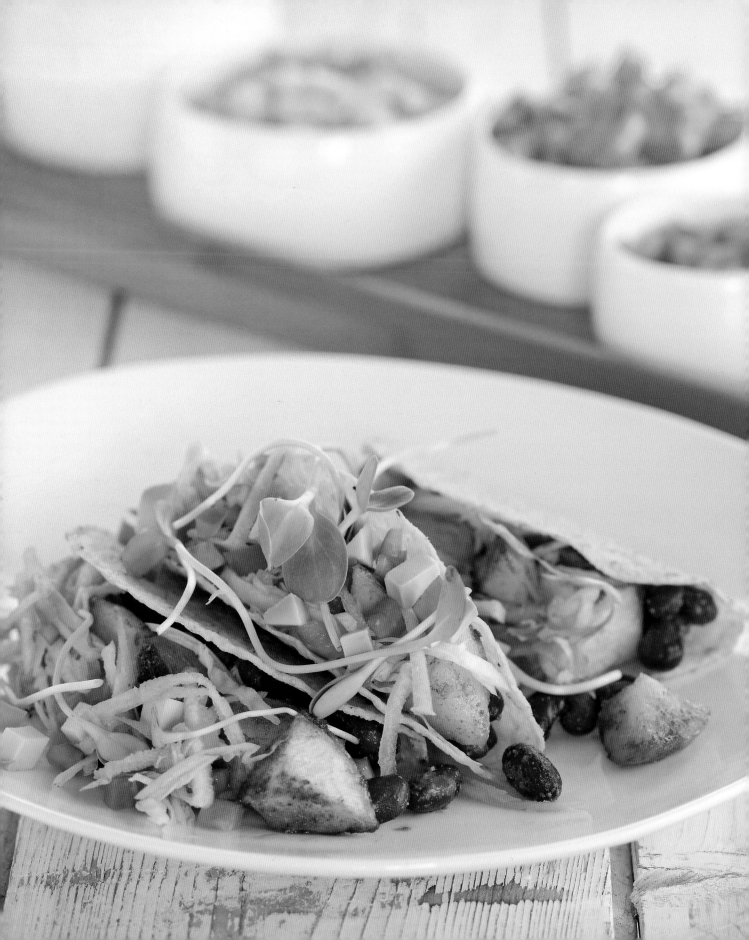

bean and potato tacos
makes 10

2 large all-purpose potatoes,
    diced
1 tablespoon olive oil
400 g (14 oz) tin red kidney
    beans, rinsed and drained
freshly squeezed juice of ½ lemon
10 taco shells
¼ small iceberg lettuce,
    shredded, to serve
3 ripe roma (plum) tomatoes,
    diced, to serve
1 carrot, grated, to serve
1 small avocado, peeled, stone
    removed and flesh diced, to
    serve
½ green capsicum (pepper),
    seeded, membrane removed
    and diced, to serve
1 small handful sunflower sprouts,
    to serve

TACO SEASONING
1 teaspoon cayenne pepper
½ teaspoon garlic powder
½ teaspoon onion powder
1 tablespoon ground cumin
½ teaspoon dry mustard
1 teaspoon sea salt
1 teaspoon paprika
½ teaspoon ground coriander

To make the taco seasoning combine all the ingredients in a small bowl and stir to combine. Store in an airtight container until needed.

Preheat the oven to 200°C (400°F/Gas 6).

Cook the potato in a saucepan of boiling water for about 10 minutes, or until just tender. Drain well, then transfer to a baking tray, drizzle over the olive oil and sprinkle over half of the taco seasoning. Bake in the oven for 20 minutes, or until golden.

Put the beans, lemon juice and remaining taco seasoning into a small saucepan over medium heat and cook for about 5 minutes, stirring often, until warmed through.

Heat the taco shells according to the packet directions. To serve, fill each taco shell with some beans, potato, lettuce, tomato, carrot, avocado, capsicum and sprouts.

tofu rice

serves 4

2 tablespoons olive oil

1 large brown onion, finely
chopped

3 carrots, thinly sliced

3 celery stalks, thinly sliced

300 g (10½ oz) firm silken tofu,
cut into 2 cm (¾ inch) dice

4 ripe tomatoes, diced

Bragg Liquid Aminos, to taste
(see note page 101)

steamed brown rice, to serve

steamed broccoli, to serve

Heat the oil in a large saucepan over medium–high heat. Add the onion and cook for about 5 minutes, or until the onion softens. Add the carrot and celery and cook for 5–7 minutes, or until softened.

Add the tofu and tomato to the pan and cook gently, uncovered, for about 15 minutes, or until the vegetables are tender. Season with Bragg Liquid Aminos, to taste. Serve with the steamed brown rice and steamed broccoli.

This was a favourite of Chloe's when she was growing up. It was not uncommon for a whole bunch of her friends to arrive at our house and this recipe is one I would throw together for a quick and easy dinner! It was a good way of getting some protein into the kids without them realising. They called it tofu rice. Funny that!

pumpkin and red lentil soup with cumin yoghurt

serves 4–6

1 kg (2 lb 4 oz) pumpkin (winter
   squash), peeled and cut into
   2 cm (¾ inch) pieces
750 g (1 lb 10 oz) orange sweet
   potato, peeled and cut into
   2 cm (¾ inch) pieces
1 large red onion, diced
200 g (7 oz) red lentils
2 litres (70 fl oz/8 cups) vegetable
   stock
2 teaspoons ground cumin, plus
   extra, to serve
250 g (9 oz/1 cup) plain yoghurt

Put the pumpkin, sweet potato, onion, lentils, stock and cumin into a large saucepan. Bring to the boil over high heat, then reduce the heat and simmer for 15–20 minutes, or until the vegetables and lentils are tender.

Remove from the heat and allow to cool slightly, then transfer to a food processor or blender and blend, in batches, until smooth. Return to the pan and heat over medium heat until warmed through. Stir through the yoghurt for a creamy consistency (or you can serve with a dollop of yoghurt on top). Divide between serving bowls and sprinkle over the extra cumin.

Tip: The yoghurt has virtually no fat compared to alternatives like coconut milk or cream, but still gives the soup a lovely smooth texture. Add more stock for a thinner consistency, or more vegetables or lentils for a thicker consistency. You can also add other vegetables, such as carrots or green peas, towards the end of cooking for added colour and texture.

A hearty soup — you should make extra so you can heat it up for a quick meal later or take it in a thermos to classes or work.

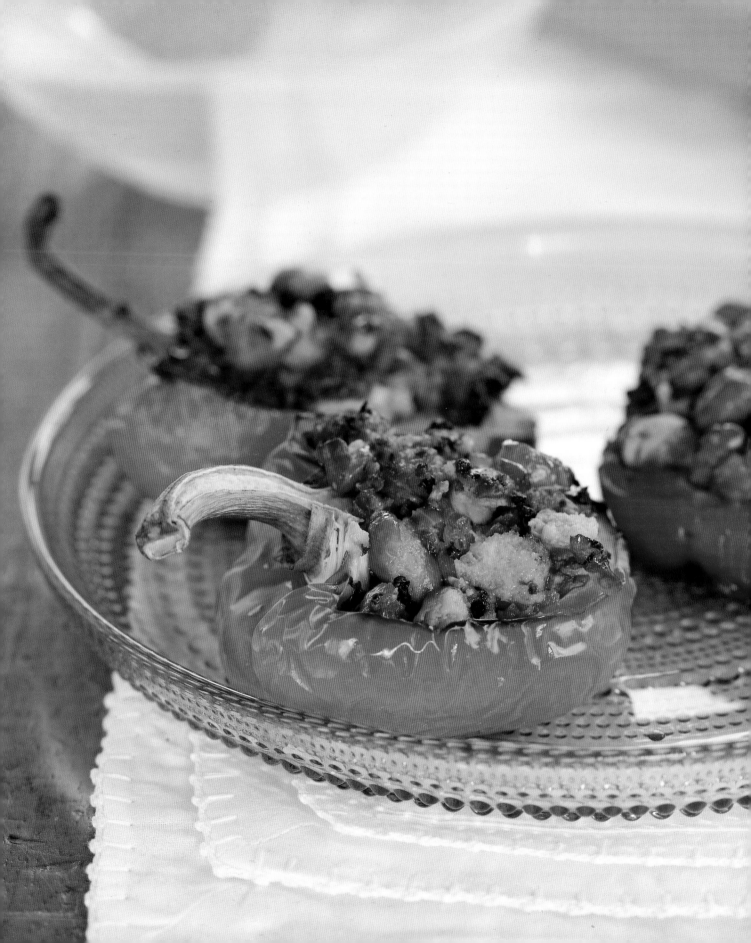

capsicums with tomato bean filling
serves 4

2 tablespoons olive oil

1 brown onion, finely chopped

2 garlic cloves, crushed

½ small eggplant (aubergine),
   finely diced

100 g (3½ oz) button
   mushrooms, finely chopped

¼ cup flat-leaf (Italian) parsley,
   finely chopped

1 tablespoon finely chopped
   oregano

4 ripe roma (plum) tomatoes,
   chopped

400 g (14 oz) tin borlotti
   (cranberry) beans, rinsed
   and drained

20 g (¾ oz/¼ cup) stale
   breadcrumbs

25 g (1 oz/¼ cup) finely grated
   parmesan cheese or vegan
   parmesan cheese (see page 76)

4 large red capsicums (peppers),
   seeded, membrane removed
   and halved lengthways, leaving
   the stalks attached

Heat 1 tablespoon of the oil in a large frying pan over medium–high heat. Add the onion and garlic and cook for about 5 minutes, stirring often, until the onion softens. Add the eggplant, mushroom, parsley, oregano and tomato. Cook for about 5 minutes, stirring regularly until the eggplant is cooked. Remove from the heat and transfer to a large bowl. Set aside to cool slightly.

Preheat the oven to 180°C (350°F/Gas 4).

Add the beans, breadcrumbs and cheese to the eggplant mixture and stir well to combine.

Brush the capsicums on the skin side with the remaining olive oil. Place the capsicum halves, cut side up, in a baking dish. Divide the bean mixture between the capsicum halves and bake for 45 minutes, or until the capsicum is tender and the filling is golden. Serve the filled capsicum with your favourite salad and dressing (see pages 80–107).

raw vegie burgers

makes 15–20

1 red onion, chopped

1 garlic clove, crushed

1 cup flat-leaf (Italian) parsley, finely chopped

¼ cup basil, finely chopped

freshly squeezed juice of 1 lemon

2 tablespoons olive oil

155 g (5½ oz/1 cup) almonds, soaked in water for 12 hours, then drained

125 g (4½ oz/1 cup) sunflower seeds, soaked in water for 6 hours, then drained

1 beetroot (beet), grated

1 red capsicum (pepper), seeded, membrane removed and finely chopped

1 zucchini (courgette), grated

1 carrot, grated

1 celery stalk, finely chopped

2 tablespoons shoyu (Japanese soy sauce)

burger buns, to serve

shredded lettuce, to serve

sprouts of your choice, to serve

sliced tomato, to serve

pesto sauce (see page 71), to serve

Put the onion, garlic, parsley, basil, lemon juice and oil in a food processor and process until smooth and combined. Add the drained almonds and sunflower seeds, beetroot, capsicum, zucchini, carrot, celery and shoyu, and process until well combined.

Shape the mixture into small round patties using ¼ cup of wet mixture. Place on plastic dehydrator sheets. Set the dehydrator temperature to high and dehydrate the patties for 4 hours. Turn the patties over and dehydrate for a further 1 hour. Remove the plastic dehydrator sheets and reduce the heat to medium. Dehydrate for 6 hours, or until patties are firm to touch .

To serve, sandwich a patty between a burger bun and layer over some lettuce, sprouts, tomato and pesto.

You will need to soak the almonds in cold water for at least 12 hours and the sunflower seeds for 6 hours before starting this recipe.

vegie sausages and homemade tomato sauce

makes 6

100 g (3½ oz/½ cup) tinned
   organic pinto beans
250 ml (9 fl oz/1 cup) vegetable
   stock
1 tablespoon olive oil
2 tablespoons shoyu (Japanese
   soy sauce)
2 garlic cloves, crushed
170 g (6 oz/1¼ cups) wheat
   gluten (see notes)
15 g (½ oz/¼ cup) nutritional
   yeast (see notes)
1 teaspoon grated fresh turmeric
½ teaspoon cayenne pepper
1 teaspoon sweet paprika
1 teaspoon dried oregano
¼ teaspoon sea salt (optional)

HOMEMADE TOMATO SAUCE
1.5 kg (3 lb 5 oz) ripe tomatoes,
   coarsely chopped
2 tablespoons olive oil
4 garlic cloves, crushed
60 g (2¼ oz/¼ cup) tomato paste
   (concentrated purée)
½ teaspoon sea salt
1 teaspoon xylitol (see note
   page 33)

To make the homemade tomato sauce, put all of the ingredients into a food processor and process until smooth. Set aside until needed. Homemade tomato sauce can be stored in an airtight container in the refrigerator for up to 3 days or frozen for up to 2 months.

Wash and drain the pinto beans well, then mash them in a large bowl until almost smooth. Add all of the remaining ingredients and stir well to combine.

Divide the mixture into six even portions and shape into 12 cm (4½ inch) logs, about 2.5 cm (1 inch) thick. Wrap each sausage in lightly-greased foil. Transfer to a bamboo steamer basket and cover with a lid.

Bring 5 cm (2 inches) water to the boil in a wok over high heat. Reduce the heat to medium, place the steamer in the wok, making sure it does not touch the water. Steam the sausages for 40 minutes, topping up the water as needed, until the sausages are cooked through.

Serve the sausages with the tomato sauce on the side.

Notes: Vital wheat gluten or gluten flour is made, as its name suggests, from the gluten of wheat. It is available from some health food stores.

Nutritional yeast, often sold as yeast flakes, is similar to brewer's yeast. It is a deactivated yeast and can be purchased at all health food stores and some large supermarkets.

balinese chicken curry
serves 4

1 tablespoon coconut oil (see
  note page 36)
500 ml (17 fl oz/2 cups) coconut
  milk
1 tablespoon grated palm sugar
  (jaggery)
2 tablespoons fish sauce
1 makrut (kaffir lime) leaf
600 g (1 lb 5 oz) chicken breast
  fillets, thinly sliced
steamed jasmine rice, to serve

CURRY PASTE

3 brown onions, coarsely chopped
4 garlic cloves, halved
8 long red chillies, seeded and
  chopped
3 cm (1¼ inch) piece fresh ginger,
  chopped
¼ cup chopped pickled galangal
  or 3 cm (1¼ inch) piece fresh
  galangal, chopped
2 tablespoons grated fresh
  turmeric
2 tablespoons finely chopped
  coriander (cilantro) root and
  stem
1 lemongrass stem, white part
  only, thinly sliced

To make the curry paste, put all of the ingredients into a food processor and process until well combined. Set aside until needed.

Heat the coconut oil in a large saucepan over medium–high heat. Scoop the coconut cream from the top of the coconut milk and add to the pan, stirring, until the oil separates from the coconut. Add the palm sugar, fish sauce and 250 g (9 oz/ 1 cup) of the curry paste and stir for 1 minute, or until aromatic. Add the coconut milk and lime leaf and bring just to the boil. Reduce the heat to medium–low and simmer, uncovered, for 10 minutes. Add the chicken and cook for 5 minutes, or until cooked through and the sauce has reduced. Serve with the steamed jasmine rice.

Note: Any leftover curry paste can be stored in an airtight container in the refrigerator for up to 4 days, or frozen for up to 3 months.

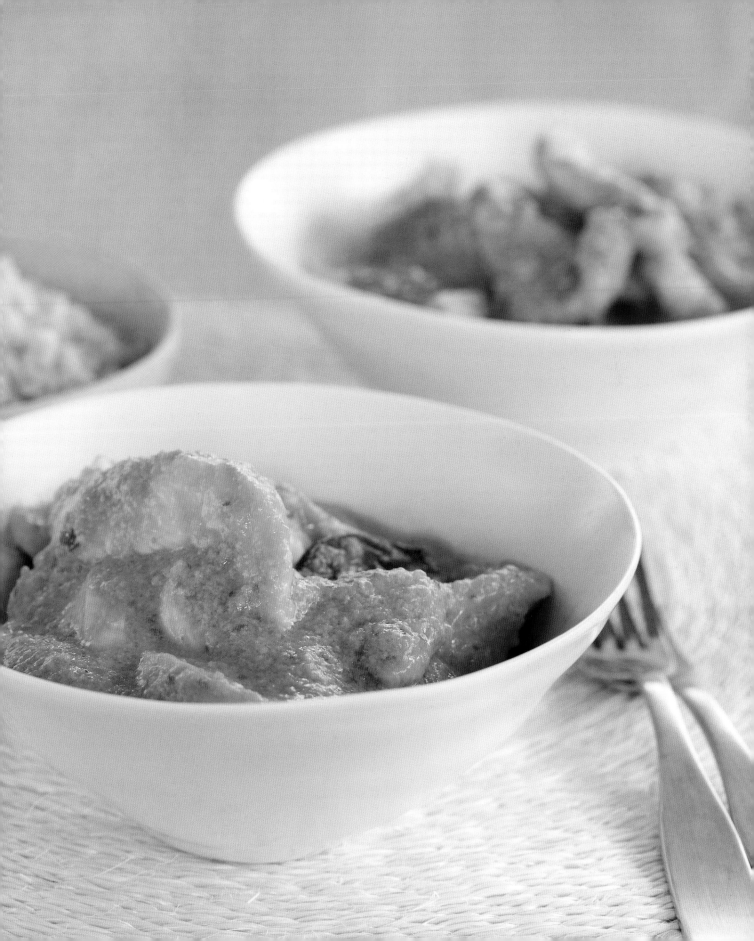

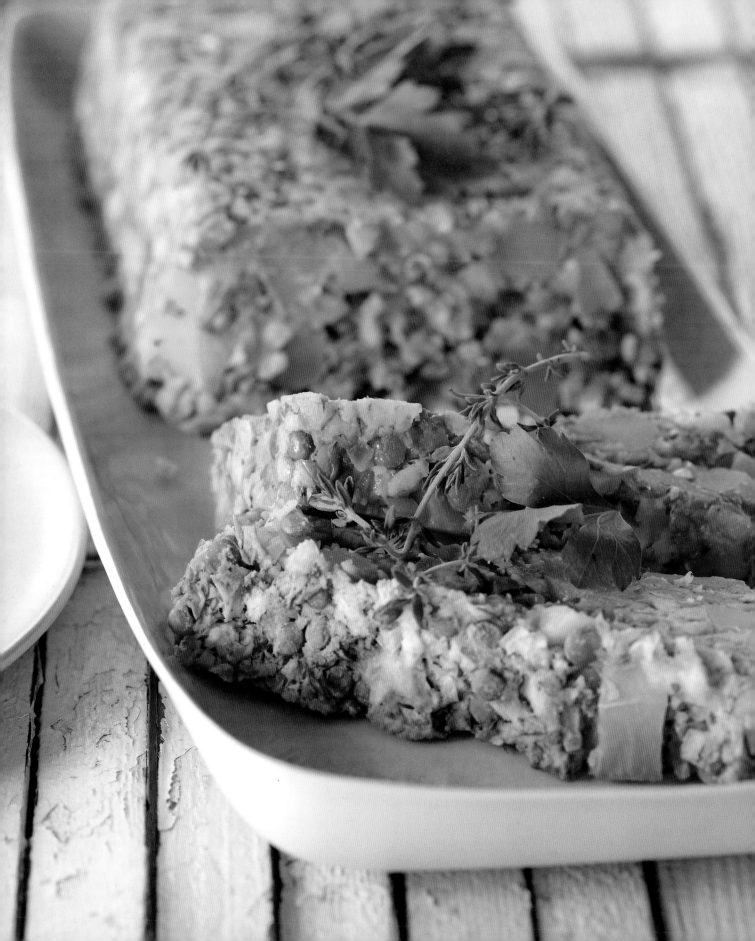

lentil and pumpkin loaf

serves 8

185 g (6½ oz/1 cup) brown lentils, rinsed

300 g (10½ oz) butternut pumpkin (squash), peeled, seeded and cut into 1 cm (½ inch) pieces

2 brown onions, finely chopped

240 g (8½ oz/3 cups) fresh breadcrumbs

2 tablespoons finely chopped flat-leaf (Italian) parsley

1 tablespoon finely chopped thyme

125 ml (4 fl oz/½ cup) full-cream (whole) milk

Preheat the oven to 190°C (375°F/Gas 5). Lightly grease a 12 x 21 x 7 cm (4½ x 8¼ x 2¾ inch) loaf (bar) tin.

Put the lentils into a saucepan, cover with water and bring to the boil over high heat. Reduce the heat and simmer for 20 minutes, or until tender. Rinse the cooked lentils under cold running water, drain well, transfer to a large bowl and set aside.

Meanwhile, cook the pumpkin in a large saucepan of boiling water for 10 minutes, or until tender. Drain and set aside.

Mash the lentils, then add the pumpkin, onion, breadcrumbs, parsley and thyme and stir well to combine. Gradually add the milk and continue stirring until the mixture just comes together.

Spoon the mixture into the prapared tin. Using the back of the spoon, press the mixture firmly into the prepared tin. Bake in the oven for 30 minutes, or until the loaf is firm to the touch. Remove from the oven and allow to cool in the tin for 10 minutes before turning out and slicing into thick slices. Serve immediately.

Tip: You can sprinkle 1 tablespoon toasted sesame seeds over the base and sides of the prepared tin before adding the lentil mixture and baking.

chicken with ginger and orange stuffing

serves 4

50 g (1¾ oz/⅔ cup) fresh gluten-
    free breadcrumbs
finely grated zest of ½ orange
½ teaspoon finely grated fresh
    ginger
1 spring onion (scallion), thinly
    sliced
½ makrut (kaffir lime) leaf, finely
    chopped
½ garlic clove, crushed
2 teaspoons finely chopped
    coriander (cilantro) leaves
1 free-range egg yolk, lightly
    beaten
4 x 165 g (5¾ oz) chicken breast
    fillets
1 tablespoon olive oil
steamed baby carrots, to serve
quinoa salad (see page 81), to
    serve

Preheat the oven to 200°C (400°F/Gas 6). Line a baking tray with baking paper.

Put the breadcrumbs, orange zest, ginger, spring onion, lime leaf, garlic, coriander and egg yolk in a bowl and mix well to combine.

Use a small sharp knife to cut a horizontal slit in the thickest part of each chicken breast to create a pocket. Divide the breadcrumb mixture into four even-sized portions and spoon into each pocket.

Heat the oil in a large frying pan over high heat. Cook the chicken for 2–3 minutes on each side, or until browned. Transfer the chicken to the prepared tray and bake for 15 minutes, or until the chicken is cooked through.

Serve the chicken breasts with the steamed carrots and quinoa salad on the side.

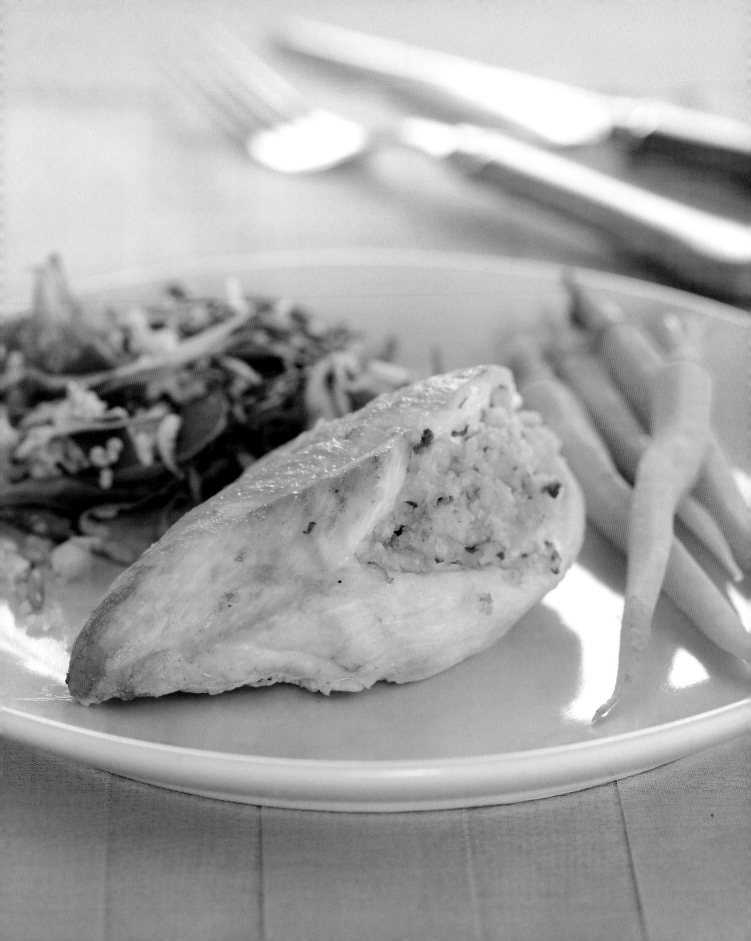

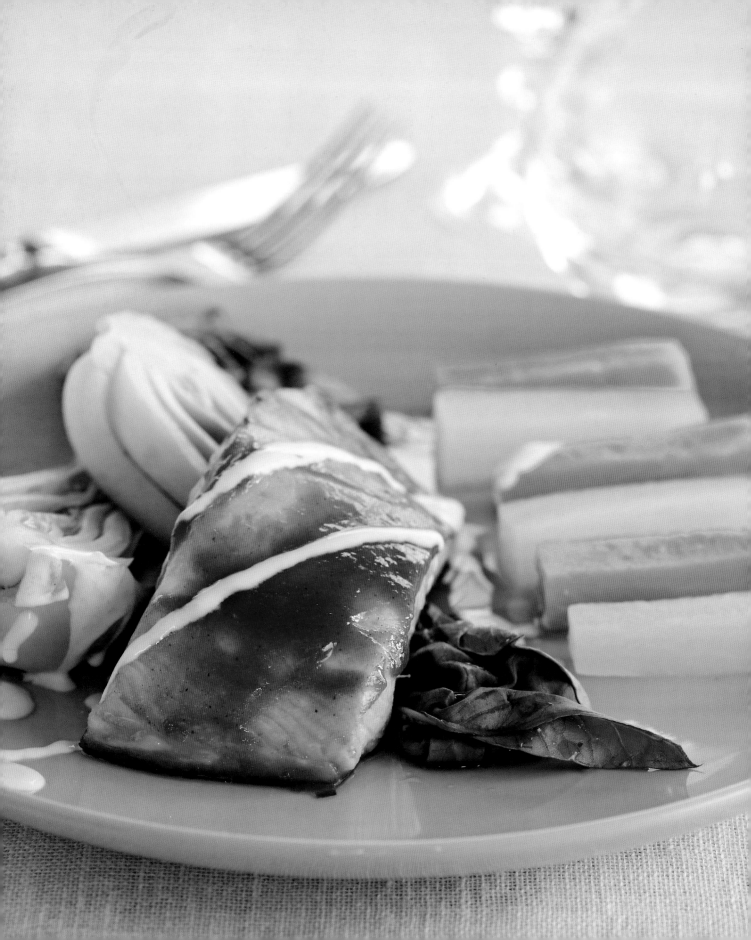

tamarind glazed salmon with wasabi yoghurt
serves 2

½ small orange sweet potato
½ small daikon radish
2 tablespoons tamarind purée
1 tablespoon mirin
1 tablespoon grated white palm
  sugar (jaggery)
pinch sea salt
1 teaspoon sunflower oil or
  light olive oil
2 x 185 g (6½ oz) salmon fillets,
  skin on
60 g (2¼ oz/¼ cup) plain yoghurt
½ teaspoon wasabi paste
2 tablespoons soy sauce
2 bok choy (pak choy), trimmed
  and halved

Preheat the oven to 180°C (350°F/Gas 4). Line a baking tray with baking paper.

Peel and cut the sweet potato into batons, each about 5 x 1.5 cm (2 x ⅝ inches) thick (try to make them as even as possible, as it adds a slight sense of formality to this dish). Repeat with the radish. Steam the potato and radish for about 12 minutes, or until tender.

Combine the tamarind, mirin, palm sugar, salt and oil in a small bowl. Place the salmon on the prepared tray and spread a heaped teaspoon of the tamarind mixture over each salmon fillet (leftover tamarind mixture will keep, covered, in the refrigerator for up to 1 week). Bake for 8–10 minutes, or until cooked through.

Meanwhile combine the yoghurt and wasabi in a small bowl.

Put the soy sauce and 60 ml (2 fl oz/¼ cup) water in a frying pan and bring to the boil. Add the bok choy and cook for 2–4 minutes, turning occasionally, or until just tender.

Arrange the sweet potato and radish batons with the bok choy on serving plates and top with the salmon fillets. Spoon a little wasabi yoghurt over the salmon and serve immediately.

This dish is contemporary Japanese in its style, it is simple to prepare, looks beautiful on the plate, and is a very delicious and healthy meal. In this dish the salmon is cooked through, and not left rare in the middle — it is a Gaia favourite.

falafels

serves 4

1 small brown onion, chopped
2 garlic cloves, chopped
¼ cup flat-leaf (Italian) parsley
freshly squeezed juice of 1 lemon
60 ml (2 fl oz/¼ cup) olive oil
1 cup sprouted chickpeas (see
    page 14)
80 g (2¾ oz/½ cup) sesame
    seeds, soaked in water for
    1 hour, then drained
155 g (5½ oz/1 cup) almonds,
    soaked in water for 1 hour,
    then drained
100 g (3½ oz/1 cup) walnuts,
    soaked in water for 1 hour,
    then drained
¼ teaspoon cayenne pepper
1 teaspoon sea salt
1½ teaspoons ground cumin
1½ teaspoons ground coriander
sprouted hummus dip (see
    page 75), to serve
tabouleh and avocado salad (see
    page 93), to serve

Preheat the oven to 180°C (350°F/Gas 4). Line a baking tray with baking paper.

Put the onion, garlic, parsley, lemon juice and oil into a food processor and process until well combined. Add the remaining ingredients and 60 ml (2 fl oz/¼ cup) water and process until well combined and the mixture comes together to form a thick paste — you may need to add a little extra water if the mixture is too dry.

Take heaped tablespoons of the mixture at a time and roll into neat balls. Repeat to make about 30 falafels in total. Place on the prepared tray and bake for 25 minutes, turning once during cooking, or until lightly browned and firm to the touch.

Serve the falafels with the sprouted hummus dip and the tabouleh and avocado salad on the side.

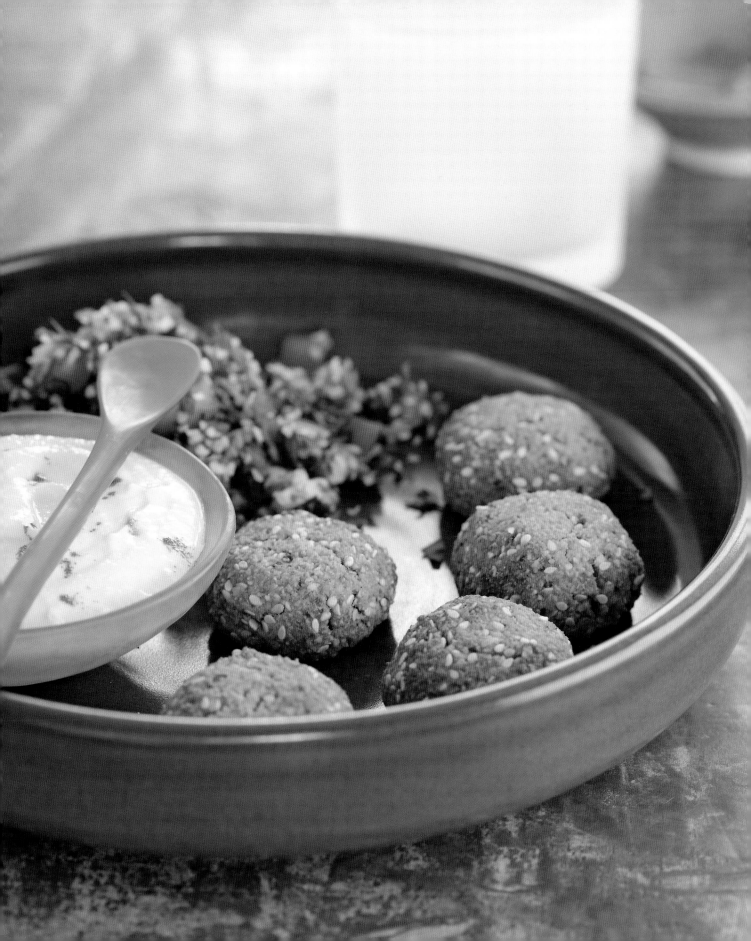

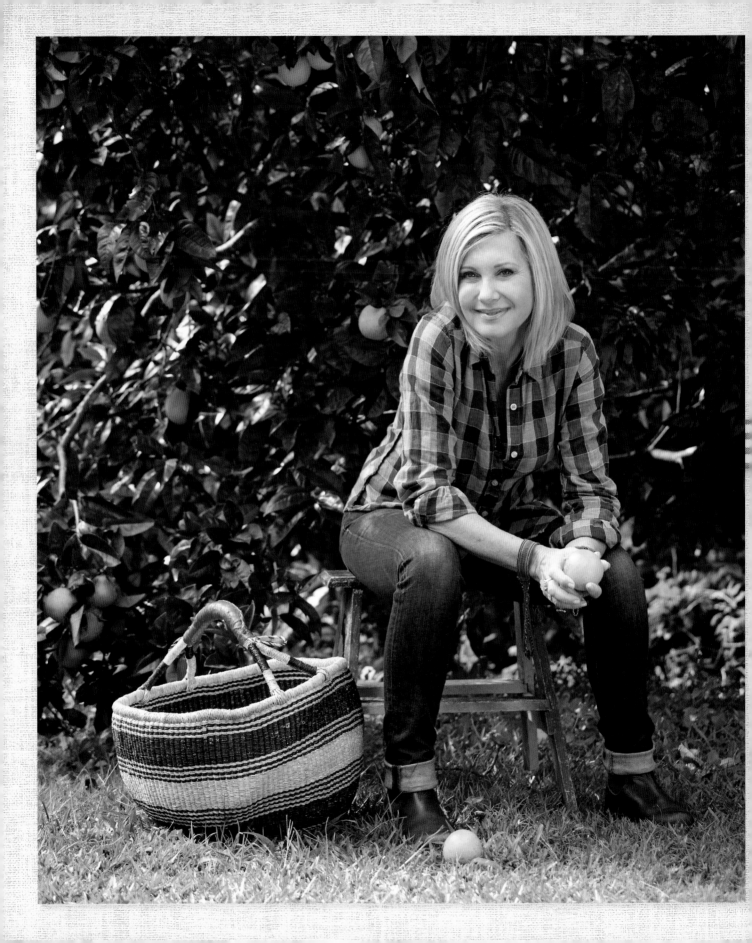

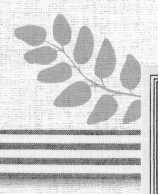

sweets

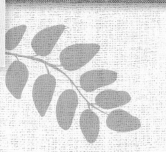

cashew, macadamia and raspberry tart

serves 8–10

25 g (1 oz/¼ cup) desiccated
   coconut
320 g (11¼ oz/2 cups) macadamia
   nuts
90 g (3¼ oz/½ cup) pitted dried
   dates, chopped

FILLING
310 g (11 oz/2 cups) cashews,
   soaked in water overnight, then
   drained
freshly squeezed juice of 1 lemon
60 ml (2 fl oz/¼ cup) agave syrup
   (see note page 22)
60 ml (2 fl oz/¼ cup) coconut oil
   (see note page 36), warmed
1 teaspoon natural vanilla extract

RASPBERRY TOPPING
250 g (9 oz/2 cups) thawed frozen
   or fresh raspberries
90 g (3¼ oz/½ cup) pitted dried
   dates, chopped

Lightly grease a round 22 cm (8½ inch) spring-form cake tin.
Line the base with baking paper and dust with the coconut.

Put the macadamias and dates into a food processor and
process until well combined. Press the date mixture over the
coconut in the base of the tin.

To make the filling, put the cashews, lemon juice, agave
syrup, coconut oil, vanilla extract and 125 ml (4 fl oz/
½ cup) water into a food processor and process until well
combined and smooth. Pour over the date mixture in the
tin. Lightly tap the tin on a work surface to remove any air
bubbles. Cover with plastic wrap and freeze for at least
2 hours, or until the filling is firm.

To make the topping, put the raspberries and dates in a food
processor and process until smooth.

Remove the tart from the tin and transfer to a serving plate.
Top with the raspberry topping and serve in wedges.

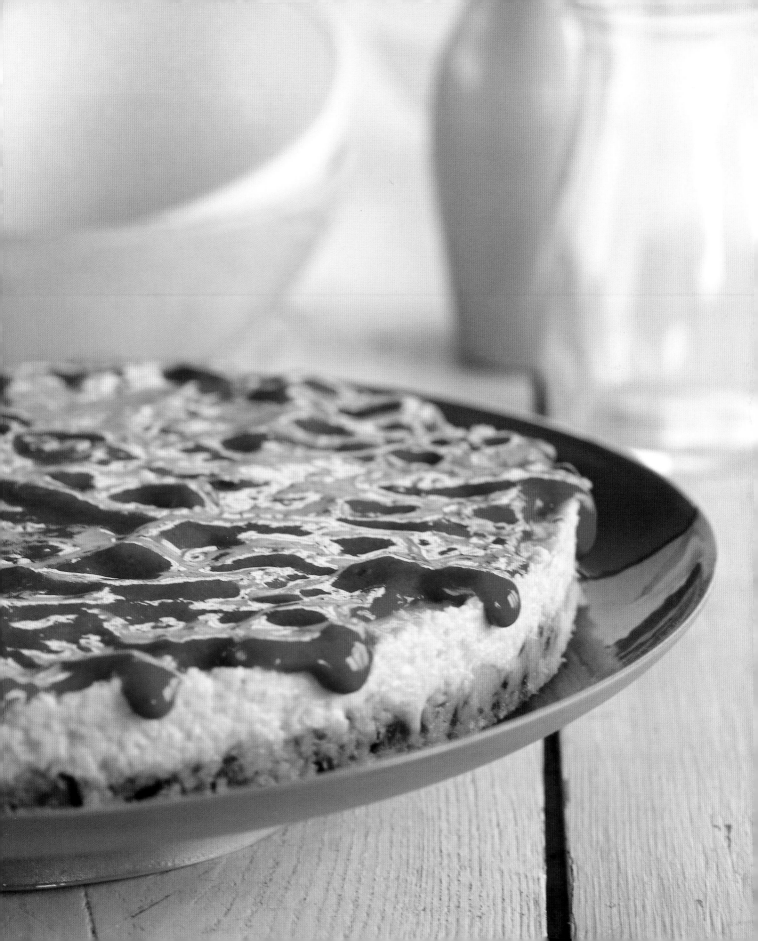

mulled pears with toasted muesli

serves 6

500 ml (17 fl oz/2 cups) red wine
100 g (3½ oz) sugar, plus extra,
    to taste
100 g (3½ oz) honey
finely grated zest of 1 lemon
finely grated zest of 1 lime
1 cinnamon stick
3 cloves
2 star anise
1 mint sprig
6 pears, peeled, halved and cored
    with stalks attached
plain yoghurt, to serve

MUESLI
100 g (3½ oz/1 cup) rolled
    (porridge) oats
30 g (1 oz/½ cup) shredded
    coconut
50 g (1¾ oz/⅓ cup) pepitas
    (pumpkin seeds)
50 g (1¾ oz) sunflower seeds
50 g (1¾ oz) flaked almonds
50 g (1¾ oz/⅓ cup) sesame seeds
pinch ground cinnamon
pinch freshly grated nutmeg

Put the wine, sugar, honey, citrus zests, spices and mint into a saucepan with 300 ml (10½ fl oz) water. Bring to the boil, then reduce the heat and simmer for 5 minutes. Add the halved pears and continue to simmer for about 45 minutes, or until the pears are tender but still holding their shape (the time will vary depending on the ripeness of the pears). Remove from the heat and leave the pears to cool in the syrup.

Preheat the oven to 200°C (400°F/Gas 6). Combine all of the muesli ingredients and spread them in an even layer on a baking tray. Cook for 6–8 minutes, or until lightly toasted.

Drain the pears and set aside. Return the cooking syrup to high heat and add the extra sugar, to taste. Bring to the boil and cook for about 5 minutes, or until it thickens. Remove from the heat and cool.

Serve the pears with a little syrup spooned over and each half sprinkled with about 1 tablespoon of the muesli. Top with a dollop of yoghurt.

Note: Any leftover muesli will keep in an airtight container for up to 2 weeks.

pear and oatmeal yoghurt muffins
makes 18

olive oil spray, for greasing

300 g (10½ oz/2 cups) plain (all-purpose) flour

3 teaspoons baking powder

½ teaspoon bicarbonate of soda (baking soda)

1 teaspoon mixed (pumpkin pie) spice or ground cinnamon

65 g (2½ oz/⅔ cup) rolled (porridge) oats

110 g (3¾ oz/½ cup) caster (superfine) sugar

2 ripe pears or apples, cored and diced with skin on

2 free-range eggs, lightly beaten

375 g (13 oz/1½ cups) mixed berry or strawberry yoghurt

125 ml (4 fl oz/½ cup) vegetable oil

Preheat the oven to 180°C (350°F/Gas 4). Lightly grease a 12-hole standard 125 ml (4 fl oz/½ cup) capacity muffin tin with olive oil spray.

Sift the flour, baking powder, bicarbonate of soda and mixed spice into a large bowl. Stir in the oats, sugar and pear.

In a separate bowl, put the egg, yoghurt and vegetable oil and stir well to combine. Add to the dry ingredients and stir until just combined.

Divide the mixture evenly between the muffin holes and bake for 15–20 minutes, or until a skewer inserted into the middle of the muffins comes out clean. Remove from the oven and turn out onto a wire rack to cool slightly. Serve warm or at room temperature.

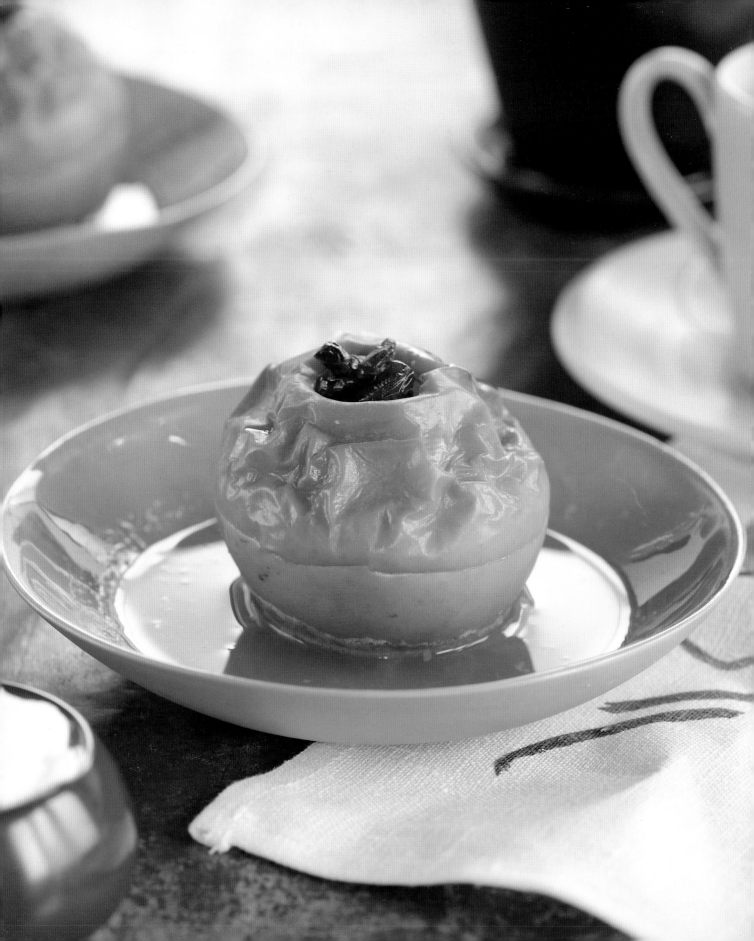

Livvy's easy baked apples
serves 4

4 apples or pears, cored

40 g (1½ oz/⅓ cup) dried fruit, such as raisins or cranberries

250 ml (9 fl oz/1 cup) freshly squeezed orange juice

2 tablespoons honey or maple syrup

plain yoghurt or ice cream, to serve (optional)

Preheat the oven to 180°C (350°F/Gas 4).

Use a sharp knife to make a shallow cut through the skin around the middle of the apple — this prevents the skin from splitting during cooking.

Place the dried fruit into the cavity of the apples and arrange the apples in a small baking dish. Pour over the orange juice and drizzle over the honey. Bake the apples for about 30 minutes, or until the juice has thickened and the apples are soft. Remove from the oven and serve warm with yoghurt or ice cream, if desired.

summer pudding
serves 6

8 slices bread, crusts removed,
  or panettone
400 g (14 oz/3 cups) fresh or
  thawed frozen mixed berries
110 g (3¾ oz/½ cup) caster
  (superfine) sugar
vanilla yoghurt, to serve

Line a 1 litre (35 fl oz/4 cup) capacity pudding basin (mould) with the bread slices, cutting them to fit the basin exactly, with a slight overlap.

Put the berries and sugar into a saucepan over medium heat. Cook very gently for 5 minutes, or until the fruit is tender. Drain the berries, reserving 125 ml (4 fl oz/½ cup) of the cooking juice.

Spoon the berries over the bread in the basin, packing it in well. Pour in the reserved juice. Arrange the remaining bread on top of the fruit in an even layer. Cover with a plate, small enough to rest on the pudding, then place a tin or other weight over the plate to weigh it down. Refrigerate overnight.

To serve, turn the pudding out of the basin and serve with vanilla yoghurt.

easy blueberry yoghurt and muesli parfait
serves 4–6

250 g (9 oz/1⅔ cups) blueberries

500 g (1 lb 2 oz/3⅓ cups)
strawberries, hulled and sliced

200 g (7 oz/2 cups) natural muesli
(see page 26)

400 g (14 oz) blueberry yoghurt

25 g (1 oz/¼ cup) flaked almonds,
toasted

Scatter half of the combined blueberries and strawberries in the base of four serving glasses. Top with a layer of muesli, then a generous dollop of yoghurt. Repeat with another layer of fruit, muesli and yoghurt, then garnish with any leftover berries and the flaked almonds.

Make this parfait when summer berries are at their peak.

panforte slice

makes about 24 pieces

200 g (7 oz) dark chocolate,
    melted
235 g (8½ oz/1½ cups) blanched
    almonds, toasted
225 g (8 oz/1½ cups) pistachio
    nuts
75 g (2½ oz/½ cup) finely
    chopped candied citrus peel
150 g (5½ oz) chopped dried
    apricots, sultanas (golden
    raisins) or figs
525 g (1 lb 2½ oz/1½ cups)
    honey, warmed
150 g (5½ oz/1 cup) plain
    (all-purpose) flour or rice
    flour, sifted
2 tablespoons raw cacao
    powder, sifted
½ teaspoon mixed (pumpkin
    pie) spice
1 teaspoon ground cinnamon

Preheat the oven to 160°C (315°F/Gas 2–3). Line an 18 x 28 cm (7 x 11¼ inch) slice tin with baking paper.

Put the chocolate, nuts, citrus peel and dried apricots in a large bowl. Stir in the warm honey until well combined.

Combine the flour, cacao powder, mixed spice and cinnamon in a separate bowl then fold through the chocolate mixture until well combined. Spread the mixture into the prepared tin and bake for 45 minutes, or until just set — the slice should be slightly moist, similar to a brownie.

Remove from the oven and allow to cool completely in the tin before cutting into portions and serving.

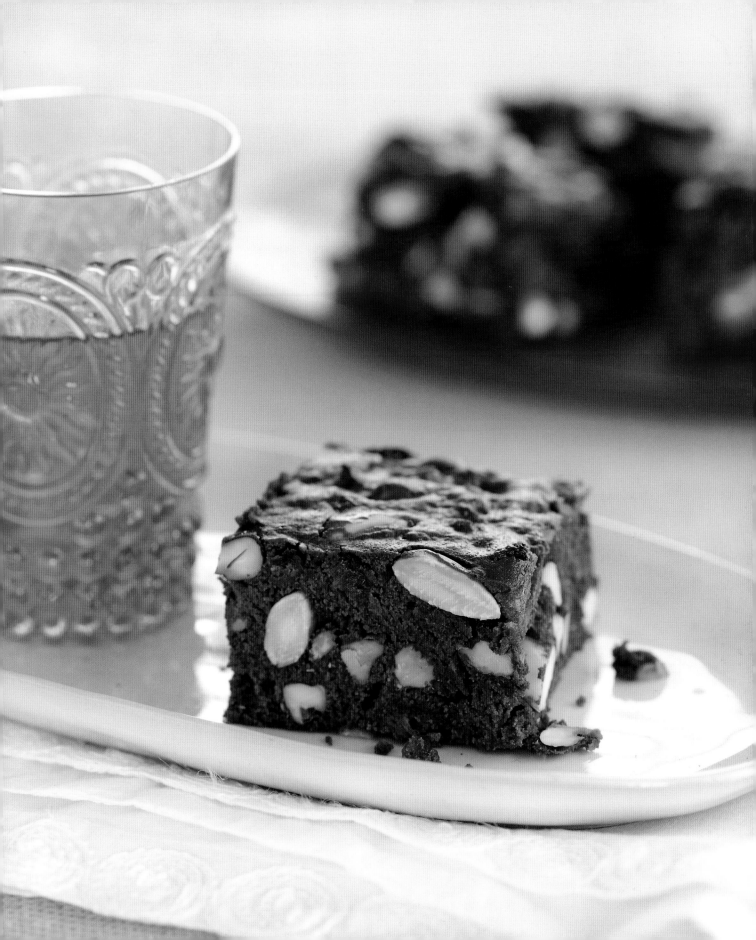

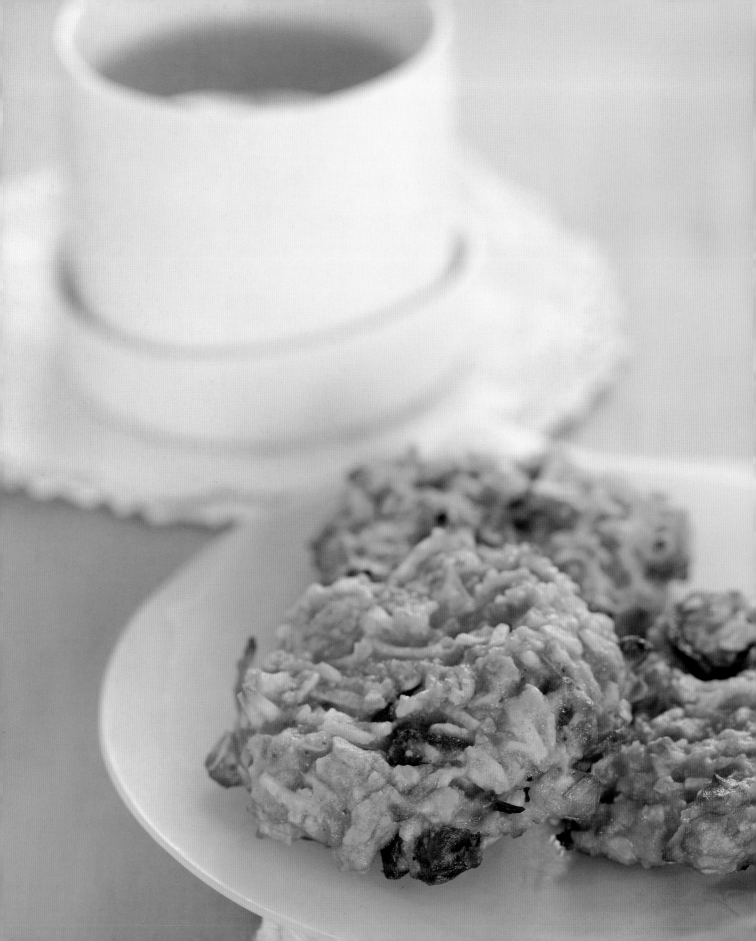

oatmeal cookies
makes 25

200 g (7 oz/2 cups) rolled
  (porridge) oats
90 g (3¼ oz/1 cup) desiccated
  coconut
150 g (5½ oz) pitted dried dates,
  chopped
250 g (9 oz/1 cup) ricotta cheese
115 g (4 oz/⅓ cup) golden syrup
3 free-range eggs
60 ml (2 fl oz/¼ cup) cold-pressed
  oil of your choice
2 large ripe bananas, mashed

Preheat the oven to 180°C (350°F/Gas 4). Line a baking tray with baking paper.

Combine the oats, coconut and dates in a large bowl.

In a separate bowl, beat together the ricotta cheese, golden syrup, eggs, oil and mashed banana until well combined. Add to the dry ingredients and stir well until the mixture holds together — if it is crumbly, add a little water, a small amount at a time, stirring well after each addition.

Drop 1 tablespoonful of the mixture at a time onto the prepared tray, leaving enough room for spreading between each one. Use a fork to flatten the mixture slightly. Bake for about 20 minutes, or until cooked through. Remove from the oven and allow to cool on the tray for 10 minutes, before transferring to a wire rack to cool completely.

The oatmeal cookies can be stored in an airtight container for up to 10 days.

Tip: Instead of dates, you can use the same quantity of drained soaked raisins, sultanas (golden raisins) or chopped dried apricots. If you like, sprinkle some sesame seeds over the top of each cookie before baking.

date and walnut truffles
makes 15–20

200 g (7 oz/2 cups) walnuts

185 g (6½ oz/1 cup) pitted dried
dates

1 tablespoon coconut oil (see
note page 36)

3 tablespoons carob powder

25 g (1 oz/¼ cup) desiccated
coconut

Put all of the ingredients except the coconut into a food
processor and process until smooth.

Take 1 teaspoon of mixture at a time and roll it into a neat
ball. Roll each truffle in coconut to evenly coat all over.
Refrigerate until ready to serve.

Note: These truffles will keep in an airtight container in the
refrigerator for up to 2 weeks. Serve at room temperature.

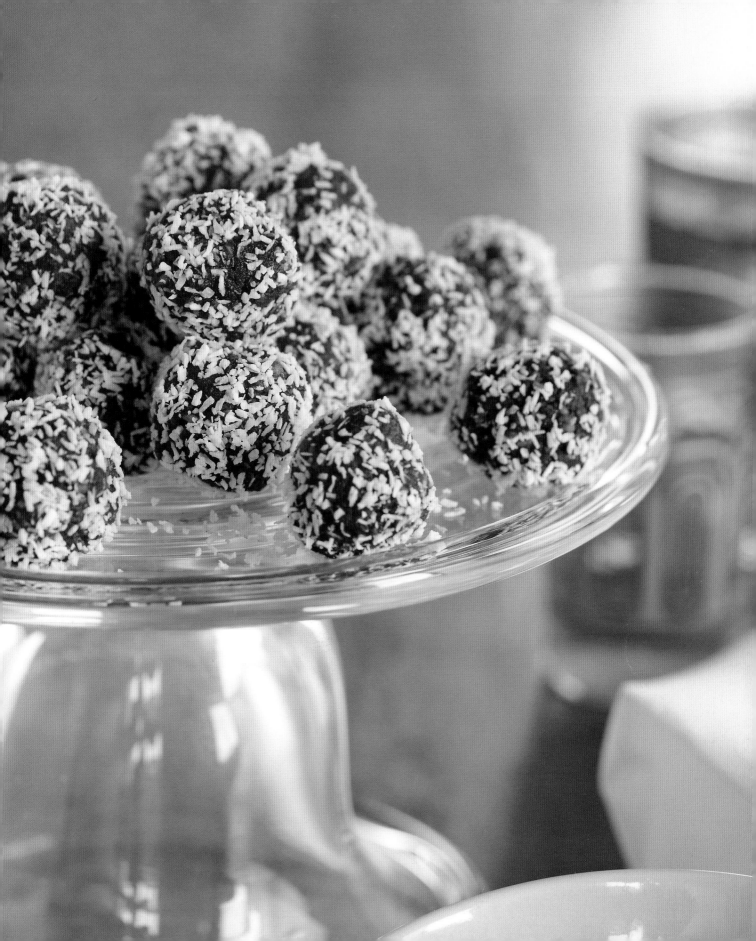

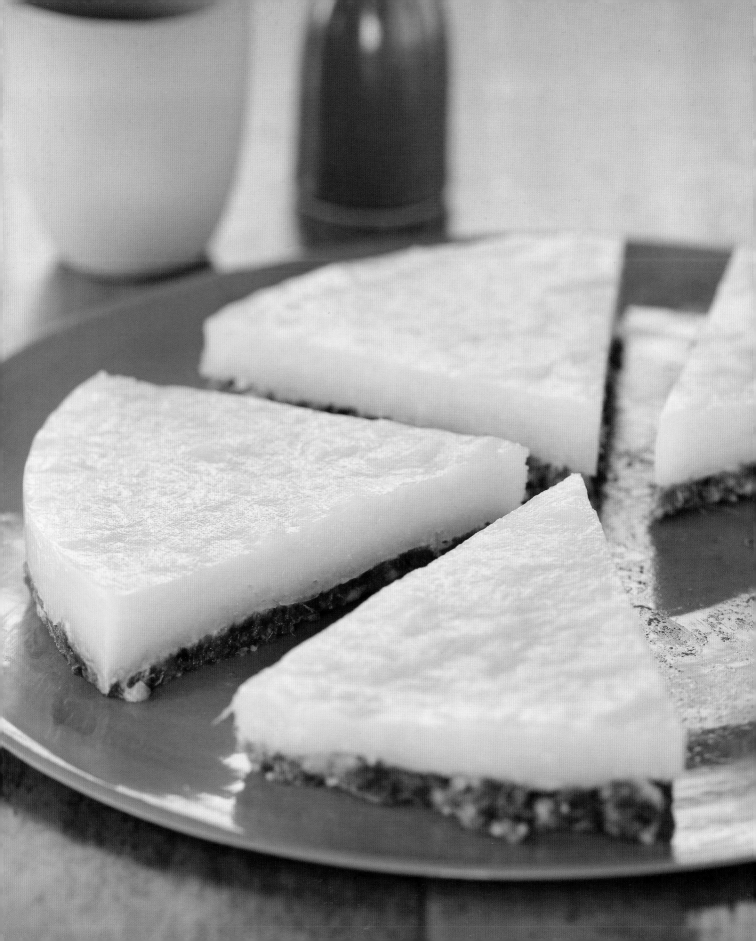

mango tart with date and macadamia crust

serves 8

2 tablespoons ground almonds

225 g (8 oz/1¼ cups) pitted dried dates

120 g (4¼ oz/¾ cup) macadamia nuts

2 teaspoons agar agar powder (see note)

2 large ripe mangoes

Lightly grease a round 20 cm (8 inch) spring-form cake tin. Dust the base with the ground almonds.

Place the dates in a heatproof bowl and pour over enough boiling water to cover. Stand for 20 minutes. Drain well and coarsely chop the dates.

Put the dates and macadamia nuts in a food processor and process until well combined. Press the date mixture in an even layer into the base of the tin.

Put 125 ml (4 fl oz/½ cup) water in a small saucepan and add the agar agar. Set aside for 5 minutes to soak. Bring to the boil over high heat, stirring. Reduce the heat and simmer gently for 3–4 minutes or until the agar agar is completely dissolved. Remove from the heat.

Peel the mangoes, remove the stones, roughly chop the flesh and place it in a blender and blend until smooth. Add the mango purée to the agar agar mixture, stirring constantly until evenly combined. Working quickly, pour the mango mixture into the tin. Cover with plastic wrap and refrigerate for at least 2 hours, or until set. Transfer to a serving plate, cut into slices and serve.

The mango tart can be stored, covered, in the refrigerator for up to 3 days.

Note: Agar agar is a natural gelling agent made from seaweed and can be used instead of gelatine. It only dissolves in boiling water. It is available from health food stores.

orange, almond and polenta cake

serves 10–12

900 g (2 lb) oranges, scrubbed

9 free-range eggs

200 g (7 oz/2 cups) ground
  almonds

175 g (6 oz) polenta

300 g (10½ oz) xylitol (see note
  page 33)

3 teaspoons baking powder

25 g (1 oz/¼ cup) flaked almonds

Put the oranges into a large saucepan and cover with water. Bring to the boil over medium heat and cook the oranges, changing the water every 30 minutes or so, for 3 hours, or until the oranges are very tender (changing the water reduces the bitterness of the peel). Refresh the oranges under cold running water and drain well. Coarsely chop the oranges, discarding any seeds and the cores.

Preheat the oven to 180°C (350°F/Gas 4). Line the base of a round 23 cm (9 inch) spring-form cake tin with baking paper.

Put the orange flesh in a food processor and process until finely chopped. Add the eggs and process until well combined. Transfer to a large bowl and stir in the ground almonds, polenta, xylitol and baking powder until combined.

Pour the mixture into the prepared tin and sprinkle the flaked almonds over the top. Bake for 1 hour–1 hour 30 minutes, or until a skewer inserted into the centre of the cake comes out clean. Remove from the oven and allow to cool in the tin for 15 minutes before transferring to a wire rack to cool completely.

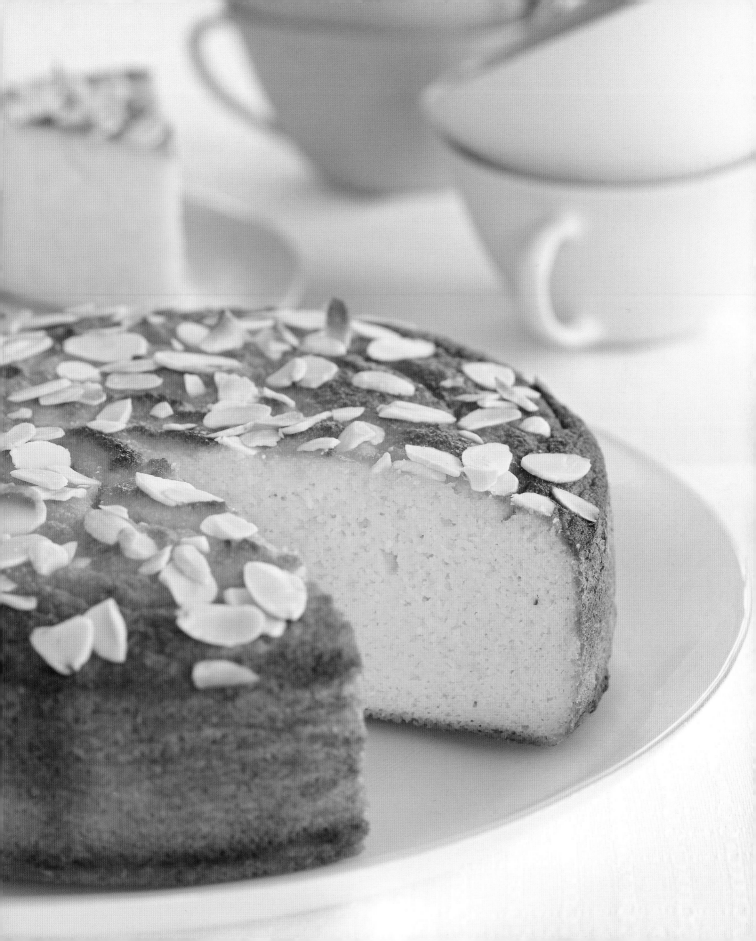

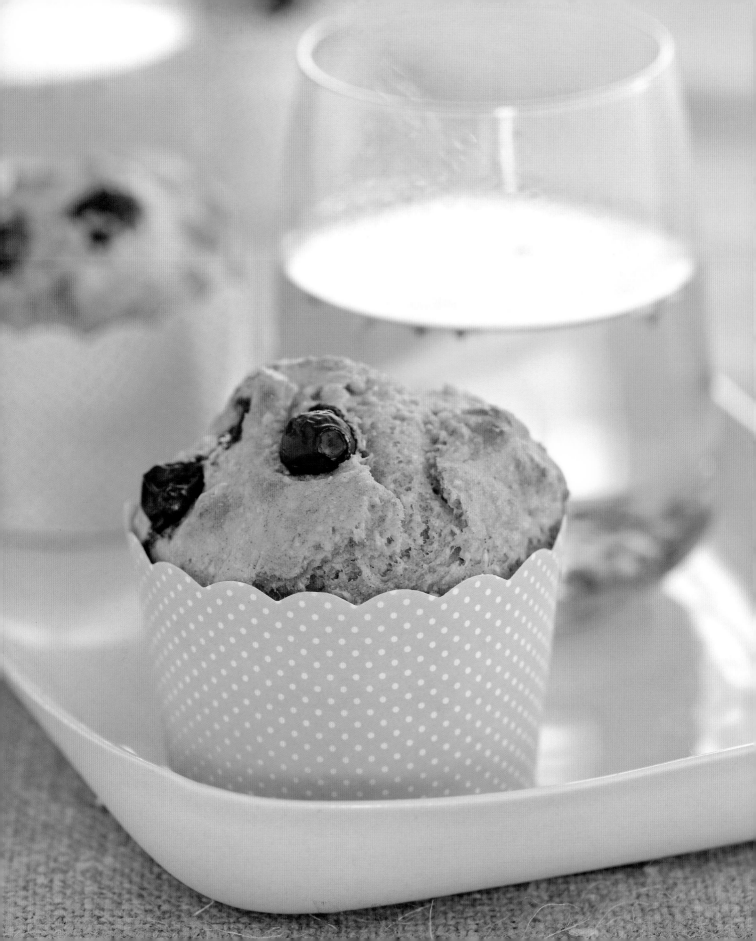

blueberry muffins
makes 12

olive oil spray, for greasing
155 g (5½ oz/1 cup) fresh or
    frozen blueberries
1 tablespoon soft brown sugar
300 g (10½ oz/2 cups) wholemeal
    (whole-wheat) self-raising flour
1 teaspoon baking powder
1 teaspoon ground cinnamon
1 free-range egg, beaten
125 g (4½ oz/½ cup) low-fat berry
    yoghurt
250 ml (9 fl oz/1 cup) low-fat milk

Preheat the oven to 210°C (415°F/Gas 6–7). Lightly grease a 12-hole standard 125 ml (4 fl oz/½ cup) muffin tin with olive oil spray or line with paper cases.

Put the blueberries and sugar in a saucepan over medium heat. Stir until the juices just start to run and the sugar dissolves. Remove from the heat and set aside to cool.

Sift the flour, baking powder and cinnamon into a bowl.

In a separate bowl, combine the egg, yoghurt and milk. Add to the dry ingredients and stir until well combined. Gently fold in the cooled blueberry mixture until combined.

Spoon the mixture evenly between the muffin holes and bake for 15–20 minutes, or until a skewer inserted into the centre of the muffins comes out clean. Remove from the oven and turn out onto a wire rack to cool.

Sometimes I use raspberries or cranberries for a change.

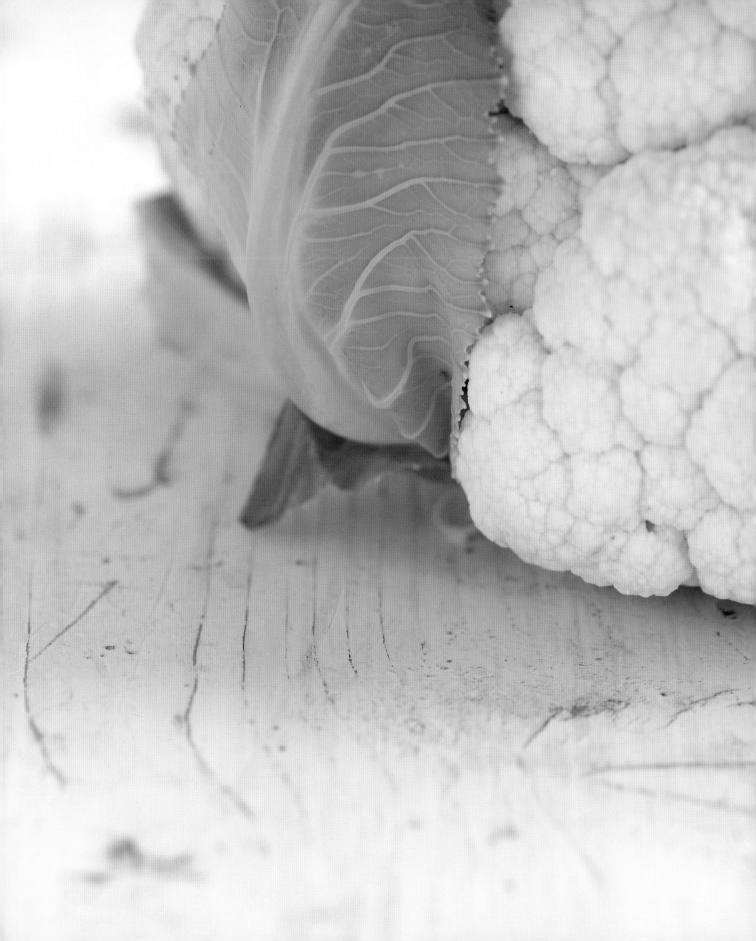

author biographies

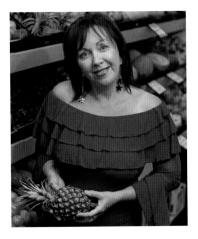

Kristine Matheson

Kristine S. Matheson was born in Sydney and is the author of bestselling book *From Cancer to Wellness: The Forgotten Secrets*. In 2005, Kristine was diagnosed with stage IV melanoma cancer and given only twelve months to live. Instead of accepting this as her fate, and with her knowledge of nutrition, strong determination, together with a positive attitude, she overcame all obstacles. Kristine became cancer-free within a few short months without any medical intervention. Kristine is passionate about treating the cause of disease and now works with her husband Wayne Matheson, regularly holding Wellness Seminars, Cancer Support Groups plus Weight Loss Challenges for charity incorporating her healthy food knowledge with Wayne's safe personal training techniques to benefit those in her community on the Gold Coast, Australia. She has been nominated for the 'Who's Who of Australian Women' award 2010–2011. For more information about Kristine Matheson go to www.cancertowellness.com or www.theforgottensecrets.com

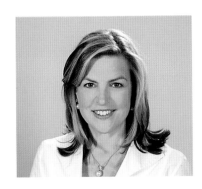

Karen Inge APD FSMA FSDA

Karen Inge is one of Australia's best-known accredited practising dietitians. She is the nutrition writer for the *Australian Women's Weekly* and regularly comments and makes appearances on radio and TV current affairs programs. She is also known for her high-profile career as a sports dietitian, working with elite athletes and developing nutrition programs for sporting organisations, as well as global food companies. An award-winning author, Karen is a sought-after speaker for her inspiring presentations to the medical and dietetic professions, corporate, education and sporting communities. She holds board positions with Jenny Craig and the Coeliac Research Fund. For more information about Karen Inge go to www.kareninge.com

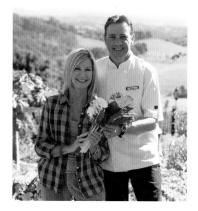

Dereck Cooper

Dereck Cooper is head chef at Gaia Retreat and Spa in Byron Bay, Australia. After taking a five-year sabbatical from his career as a chef, Dereck decided to work in the neurological field and learnt a lot about the amazing benefits food can have on mind, body and soul. Returning to the kitchen with renewed enthusiasm, Dereck now embraces a holistic approach to cooking — using food as a medicine.

Leah Roland

Founding Principal of the Bangalow Cooking School Leah has also run a catering business in Sydney and published many food articles in Australia. She has implemented a health and lifestyle cooking program at The Buttery, a leading drug and alcohol rehabilitation facility in Binna Burra, NSW, and placed educational food programmes in many regional schools. Leah has now joined the Gaia team as a chef where she relishes the holistic approach to fundamentally good food.

Campbell Rowe

Born and raised on an Olive orchard in the Wairarapa, New Zealand, Campbell moved to Australia after completing his chef training in 1999. Taking a position at Yandina's Spirit House restaurant on The Sunshine Coast, he developed a love for Thai and Asian-inspired cuisine. He eventually moved to the Byron Shire to study organic farming in production horticulture at Wollongbar Primary Industries Institute. After qualifying in 2008, he took a traineeship on an organic farm to help establish a 6000 hen free-range egg operation. He is currently employed as Gaia's sous chef and enjoying working with fresh produce from the organic garden.

Toni Golds

Toni has been working at Gaia Retreat and Spa for three years. She is also studying at the Wollongbar TAFE Northern Rivers NSW.

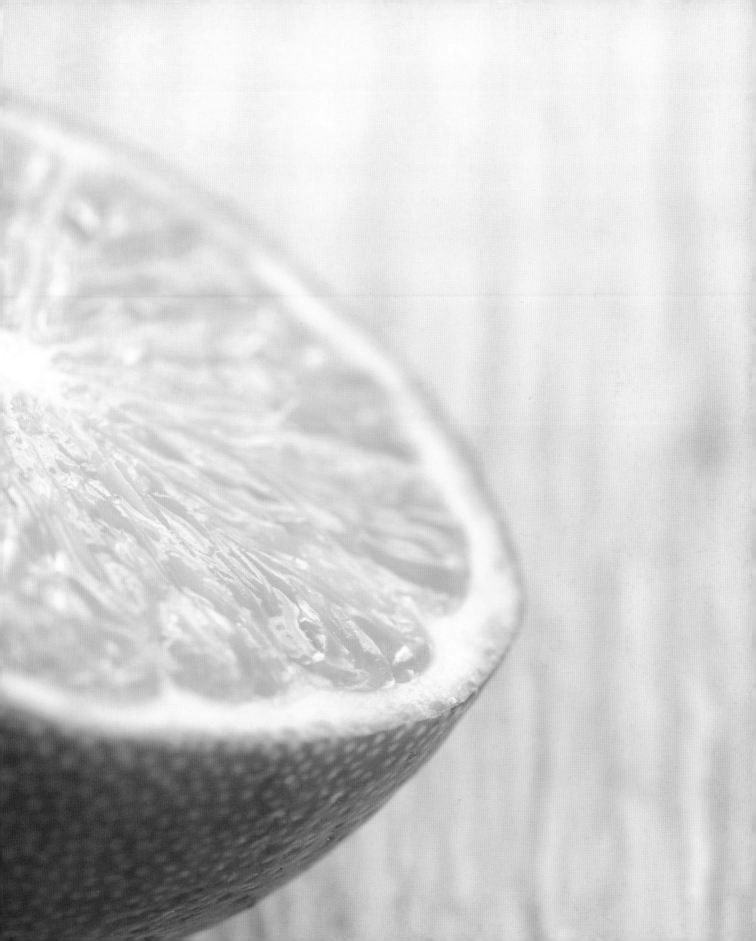

index

Published in 2011 by Murdoch Books Pty Limited

Murdoch Books Australia
Pier 8/9
23 Hickson Road
Millers Point NSW 2000
Phone: +61 (0) 2 8220 2000
Fax: +61 (0) 2 8220 2558
www.murdochbooks.com.au

Murdoch Books UK Limited
Erico House, 6th Floor
93–99 Upper Richmond Road
Putney, London SW15 2TG
Phone: +44 (0) 20 8785 5995
Fax: +44 (0) 20 8785 5985
www.murdochbooks.co.uk

Publisher: Kylie Walker
Photographer (Food): Natasha Milne
Photographer (Olivia and cover): Michele Aboud
Stylist: Jody Vassallo
Project Manager: Livia Caiazzo
Editor: Jacqueline Blanchard
Designer: Tania Gomes
Production: Joan Beal

National Library of Australia Cataloguing-in-Publication Data:

Author: Newton-John, Olivia, 1948-
Title: LivWise / Olivia Newton-John.
ISBN: 9781742662251 (Australia)
ISBN: 9781742666754 (UK)
Notes: Includes index.
Subjects: Cooking (Natural foods)
             Diet therapy--Australia.
Dewey Number: 641.563

A catalogue record for this book is available from the
British Library.

IMPORTANT: Those who might be at risk from the effects
of salmonella poisoning (the elderly, pregnant women,
young children and those suffering from immune deficiency
diseases) should consult their doctor with any concerns
about eating raw eggs.

OVEN GUIDE: You may find cooking times vary depending
on the oven you are using. For fan-forced ovens, as a
general rule, set the oven temperature to 20°C (35°F) lower
than indicated in the recipe.

RECIPE CONTRIBUTORS:
Kristine Matheson: pages 25, 26, 30, 33, 34, 35, 36, 45, 50,
52, 53, 54, 59, 60, 64, 70, 71 (bottom), 72, 75, 76, 77, 82, 89
(bottom), 91, 98, 102, 120, 123, 129, 130, 134, 141, 150, 151
(top),164, 176, 180.
Toni Golds: pages 22, 29, 39, 81, 115
Todd Cameron: pages 159, 179
Campbell Rowe: page 85
Michael Jennings: page 90
Leah Roland: pages 93, 94, 102 (bottom), 105 (top), 160, 172
Dereck Cooper: pages 68, 71 (top), 111, 112, 124, 142,
152, 156
Karen Inge: pages 27, 40, 41, 52 (bottom), 85 (top), 107
(top), 118, 119, 126, 127, 155, 166, 167, 170, 171, 175

The publisher and stylist would like to thank
the following:

Top3bydesign - www.top3bydesign.com.au
Mud Australia - www.mudaustralia.com
Design Mode International - www.iittala.com
Robert Gordon - www.robertgordonaustralia.com
Spotlight - www.spotlight.com.au/
Bison - www.bisonhome.com/
Lucy Vanstone ceramics - http://vanstoneceramic.
squarespace.com/wheel-of-life-studio/
Dinosaur Designs - www.dinosaurdesigns.com.au/
Parterre Garden - http://www.parterre.com.au/
Gaia Retreat and Spa - http://www.gaiaretreat.com.au/

Printed by 1010 Printing International Limited, China
Reprinted 2011 (twice)